If Only I'd Known That A Year Ago...

*Everything you need to know about living with
ill health, injury or disability*

Published by RADAR PROMOTIONS LTD for

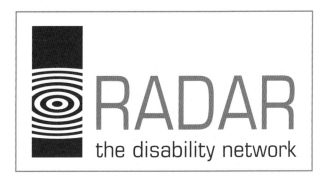

Registered Charity Number 273150

**THE ROYAL ASSOCIATION
FOR DISABILITY RIGHTS**

**12 City Forum
250 City Road
London EC1V 8AF**

☎ **020 7250 3222**
F **020 7250 0212**
Minicom **020 7250 4119**

**Edited by
John Stanford**

**8th Edition
ISBN 978-0-9561995-6-0**
© **RADAR PROMOTIONS LTD 2010**

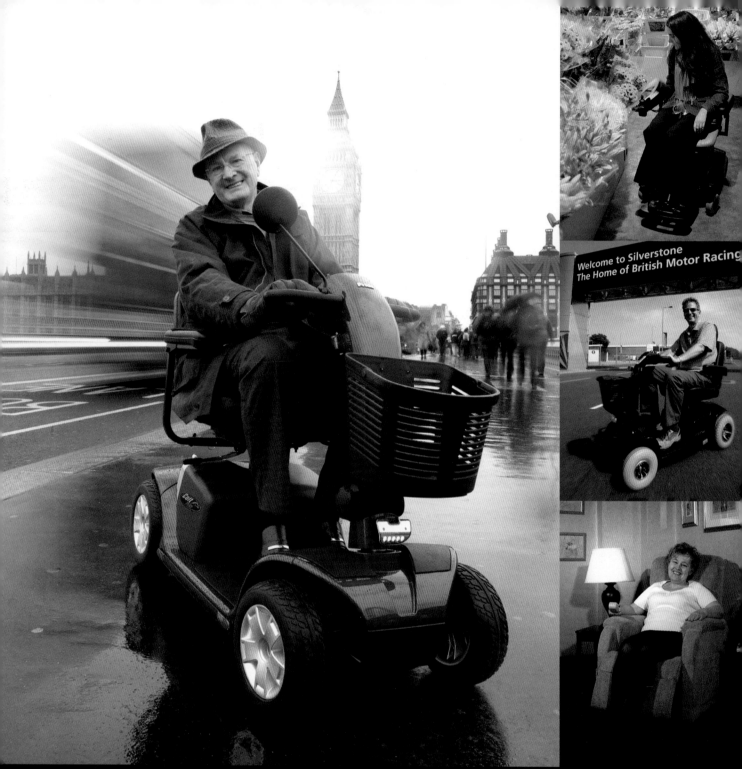

Live Life to the Full with Pride

Scooters, Power Chairs, Lift and Recline Chairs and more; Pride stands for the best in quality, reliability, comfort and style. Designed to be easy to use, Pride produces mobility products to help you live your life to the full.
Our wide range means finding the right choice to suit your life style has never been easier.
Call Pride to find your nearest dealer or take a look at our web site for more details.

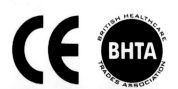

Pride
Mobility Products Ltd

Pride Mobility Products Ltd. T: 01869 324 600 F: 01869 323 070 www.pridemobility.com

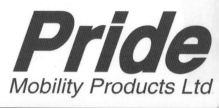

Publisher
Adrian Chance
rpl@radar.org.uk

Sales & Production coordinator
Marriott Lusengo

Design
**Marriot Lusengo &
Segun Omotuyole**

Printed by
Cambrian Printers
Lianbadarn Road
Aberystwyth Dyfed SY23
01970 627 111
www.cambrian-printers.co.uk

Cover images

"Agus Yusuf, mouth painter."
Source/Photographer Sofwan Ardyanto

"Dutch disabled dancers."
Photographer Viktor Drachev
Picture Library: Getty

"Autistic child at an indoor play centre"
Copyright Duncan Phillips
Picture Library: Reportdigital

Bharatanayam on Wheels
Ability Unlimited India

**"Family of four sits outside on a sunny
summer day for a portrait."**
Photographer Rhea Anna
Picture Library: Getty

RADAR

Foreword

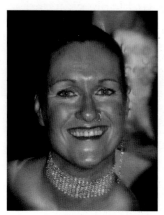

Alison Lapper

Whether you are recently disabled, or have been diagnosed with a long-term mental or physical health condition, or have a disabled child or other relative – this book answers the questions constantly asked by people in exactly those situations. It also answers questions posed by people like me, disabled from birth.

The answers are specific – from benefits to mental health support, from employment advice to housing adaptations and travel (and much more). But the purpose is wider: to enable everyone living with ill-health, injury or disability to lead the life that we want to lead. Information - and experience from others who have trod the path before - helps us all achieve that. And this isn't an occasional experience. No less than one in five of us has a long-term impairment or health condition that would be considered a 'disability' under the legislation that protects us from discrimination. Add to that our involvement with relatives, friends and colleagues who experience disability and we are all touched by the experience.

For me – born without arms in a society that saw that as abnormal – I was brought up to use prosthetic limbs and 'fit in'. But, drawing on the experience of other disabled people, I took a different path as I developed both as an artist and as a mother. Photographs of me with my baby son challenged old notions that there is one 'normal' model of parenting or that disabled people cannot successfully raise children. My art questions notions of physical normality and beauty and questions whether 'disability' can evoke more than revulsion, pity or sympathy.

This book provides the information you need at important moments in life, to enable you to seize that equality of opportunity, for instance:

- ❯ after an accident
- ❯ when you receive a diagnosis (from multiple sclerosis to bi-polar disorder, epilepsy or dementia)
- ❯ when a disabled child is born
- ❯ when a long-standing impairment enters a new phase or
- ❯ when other circumstances change – from redundancy to becoming a parent.

Life can seem strange and confusing. The life you expected has suddenly changed. Many millions of people have been through this process and come through the other side. Life may not be as it was before, but as you go through your own process of recovery you often find you can negotiate for changes (supports with your family life, adjustments at work – and more) that give you choice and control - give you your life back. Every experience is different; but the common thread is that we can choose how to lead our lives if we have the information and support to create our own life journey. This book can guide you on your way.

Since some services are very local, and change rapidly, this guide cannot be completely comprehensive – but it is packed with information that I hope you will find helpful.

Alison Lapper, MBE
March 2010

Britain's train companies working together to make rail travel easier

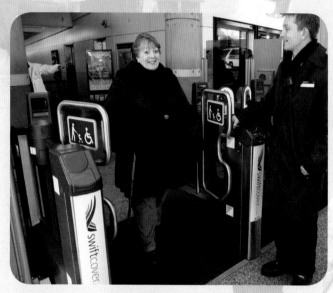
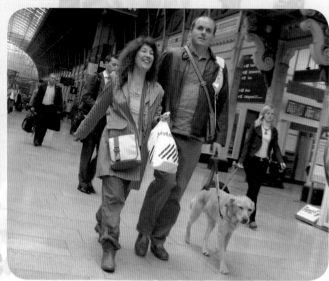
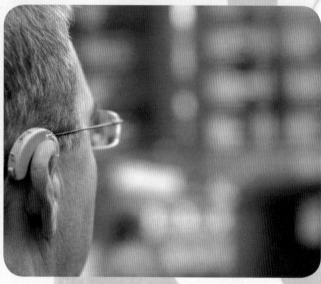
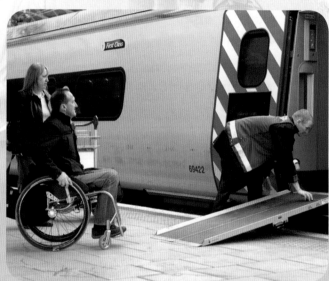

Stations made easy →

Check out the new 'Stations Made Easy' journey planning application at:

www.nationalrail.co.uk/stations_destinations

or call 08457 48 49 50 to arrange assistance for your journey

For more information on how to save money when you travel see **www.disabledpersons-railcard.co.uk**

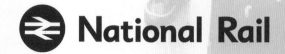
National Rail

INTRODUCTION

RADAR provides a national voice to people living with ill health, injury or disability in the UK. We draw on a wide range of experiences to inform Government, Parliament and major national organisations. We believe disabled people should be able to participate in every aspect of life. Making sure that people have the skills, jobs and support they and their families need is important for everyone – from the younger person enabled to stay, and progress, at work to the older person with the support they need to sustain the activities and relationships that matter to them (and to their families and friends). RADAR has the solutions that can make the UK work better for everybody – from designing accessibility into housing and transport from the outset; to stripping away outdated and prejudiced attitudes that can hold people back.

RADAR (Royal Association for Disability Rights) is led by people with direct personal experience of disability or health conditions. We have over 400 organisational members. We support disabled people's leadership and empowerment: for instance, in 2010 we are supporting 100 disabled people to pursue their leadership ambitions and make a difference, from being a school governor to influencing social care or developing the career or their choice.

In the last year we have made important national policy gains. We influenced Government to improve the Access to Work scheme (increasing the budget and making it better for people with fluctuating conditions). We influenced the Equality Bill, to make sure nothing was lost from the Disability Discrimination Act and that there were new rights: no pre-employment health checks before job offer (to rule out unfair job discrimination); and new rights for disabled children to auxiliary aids at school.

To join RADAR and receive regular updates email radar@radar.org.uk or call 020 7250 3222. To find out about RADAR's other guides and campaigns call us or go to http://radar-shop.org.uk

We welcome feedback on this book so we can continually improve it. Please contact email rpl@radar.org.uk

Liz Sayce, OBE
Chief Executive
March 2010

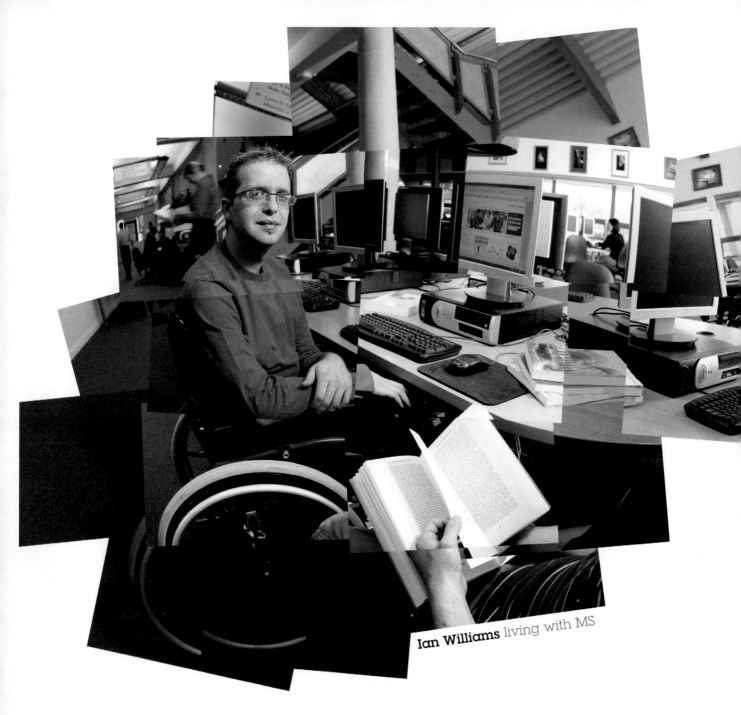

Ian Williams living with MS

"Have you still got MS?"
"Yes, I've got it for life. There's no cure."

No one knows what causes MS and they've yet to find a cure. But with the MS Society's support, I have a rich and fulfilling life. They've got a freephone helpline **0808 800 8000** and you can visit **www.mssociety.org.uk** to find out more or make a donation.

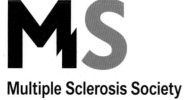

Multiple Sclerosis Society

MS Society. Putting the pieces together.

The Multiple Sclerosis Society of Great Britain and Northern Ireland is a charity registered in England and Wales (207495) and Scotland (SC016433)

ADVOCACY AND DECISION MAKING

Advocacy

Sometimes the social care, benefits, welfare rights or health care system can seem an impenetrable maze, especially if you are new to it all. It's worth remembering though that many disabled people have been through and understood how the "system" works.

Equally, many disabled people, who have fought hard to understand and exercise their rights, have formed organisations to support people struggling to manage their rights, largely through lack of knowledge and experience. As supporters of "advocacy" these groups are often referred to.

The very word "advocacy" can mean different things to different people. We've defined advocacy here as a way of supporting disabled people to speak up, get what they are entitled to and retain or regain an independent life.

Advocacy, ideally, will mean supporting and educating you so that you can speak up for yourself. It can also mean being with you as you navigate statutory systems or even, if you choose, speaking on your behalf.

The best way to secure a local advocacy service is to follow one or more of the following tips:

❯ Contact the National Centre for Independent Living (NCIL). They may well know of a Centre for Independent Living close to you that runs an advocacy service. (Contact details can be found in the Independent Living chapter.)

❯ Contact a large, national, impairment or subject related charity that's relevant to you. Again, they may know of a local service that's appropriate to you. Examples of these organisations include Age Concern, the MS Society, RNID, RNIB, MIND and so on. (Contact details can be found in the Useful Contacts chapter.)

Power of Attorney

There may be a time in the future when you think things might get difficult and you might struggle to manage your day to day affairs. It's crucial to attend to the future whilst you easily can. Tackling the issue now means that you will nominate people – friends, relatives, supporters and so on – who you really trust to help you.

The law on this subject is complex and has recently changed. The new law is called the Mental Capacity Act. When the Bill was being discussed in the Houses of Parliament it was originally called the Mental Incapacity Bill. So strong was disabled peoples organisations' view of the word "incapacity" – making assumptions about disabled people's inability to deal with matters – that the name of the law was changed and the theme of capacity was embodied within the Act.

So, the Mental Capacity Act now means that, in all cases, those with whom you deal must always assume you have the capacity to make a decision.

You can, however, use the law to write a legal document that will enable you to legally trust someone you name and who is willing to act on your behalf in certain, specific circumstances.

You can write this document well in advance of ever needing to use it. Just because you've written the papers doesn't mean they are immediately in force – you might never use them. Essentially, you are insuring yourself for the future and will only "claim" when you need or want to.

The Government Department that deals with Power of Attorney is called the Office of the Public Guardian – the OPG. The OPG is there to make sure that people's best interests are always guarded and supported. The OPG maintains a helpful website, which is packed with essential detail about these powers.

What follows is a very brief overview of an extremely complex area of law. It is possible for an individual to draft the majority of a Lasting Power of Attorney, but the best advice will always be a consultation with either your advocacy group or a solicitor.

A Lasting Power of Attorney (LPA) is a legal document that you (the Donor) make using a special form. It allows you to choose someone now (the Attorney) that you trust to make decisions on your behalf about things such as your property and affairs or personal welfare at a time in the future when you no longer wish to make those decisions or you may lack the mental capacity to make those decisions yourself.

An LPA **can only be used** after it is registered with the Office of the Public Guardian (OPG).

There are two different types of LPA - **a Personal Welfare LPA** and **a Property and Affairs LPA.**

You can get detailed guidance on LPAs in the guidance booklets section of the OPG's website.

Anyone aged 18 or over, with the capacity to do so, can make an LPA, appointing one or more Attorneys to make decisions on their behalf. You cannot make an LPA jointly with another person; each person must make his or her own LPA.

The following are the different people involved in making an LPA:

The Attorney(s). An Attorney is the person(s) you choose and appoint, using an LPA form, to make decisions on your behalf about either your personal welfare or property and affairs or both. It is an important role and one that the person chosen has to agree to take on. If you were to register the LPA in the future, depending on which type it is, your attorney could, for instance, pay bills from your personal bank account on your behalf; they could negotiate and agree a direct payment with your local Social Services Department; they could agree to medical or surgical intervention. But they must always act in your best interests and will be regulated as doing so by the Office of the Public Guardian.

A Donor is someone who makes an LPA appointing an Attorney(s) to make decisions about his/her personal welfare, property and affairs or both.

A **named person** is someone chosen by the Donor to be notified when an application is made to register their LPA. They have the right to object to the registration of the LPA if they have concerns about the registration. The named person(s) are specified in the LPA form. Selecting people to notify of an application to register is one of the key safeguards to protect you if you make an LPA.

A **certificate provider** is a person the Donor must select to complete a Part B Certificate in the LPA form. The certificate provided must confirm that the Donor understands the LPA and that the Donor is not under any pressure to make it. The certificate provider is another important safeguard.

A **witness** is someone who signs the LPA form to confirm that they witnessed:

> the Donor (the person making the LPA) signing and dating the LPA form; or

> the Attorney(s) (the person appointed by the Donor) signing and dating the LPA form.

It is an important role and acts as a further safeguard.

To summarise:

> Making a Lasting Power of Attorney now is always a good idea

> You should always involve someone trained or qualified to advise you

> Making an LPA does not mean it is immediately active – you need never use it if you so choose

> When you want to enact the content of an LPA, it must be registered with the Office of the Public Guardian.

Office of the Public Guardian

Archway Tower, 2 Junction Road, London N19 5SZ.
☎ 0845 330 2900. Textphone: 020 7664 7755. Ⓦ www.publicguardian.gov.uk

Advance Directives

A will is a statement by an individual giving their instructions on how, typically, property and money should be dealt with after death. Other matters such as funeral and burial arrangements may be incorporated.

Whereas ordinary wills have been used for centuries the concept of an 'advanced directive' is relatively new. Concerns about mental capacity and consent for treatment have become more of an issue with medical advancement and interventions such as cardiopulmonary resuscitation, artificial ventilation and intravenous hydration and nutrition. Some people become concerned about having treatment when incapable of refusing treatments or when they are unable to consent or incapable of consenting. A person may make a will or advance directive to the effect that in such circumstances they would not wish to be subjected to medical intervention.

RADAR believes people should be able to specify in advance that they do want treatment if they become unable to decide at a later date, as well as to state that they do not want treatment. Some forms in use for advanced statements enable you to do this. This does not have legal force but may be taken into account, so it is worth doing if it is your wish to do so.

Problems can arise with the practical definition, application and implementation of such directives. Often the request for such a directive to be put in place can provide a useful opportunity to discuss current or future illness with family and friends.

The creation of an advance directive with a focus on the denial of medical intervention in certain events is an extremely serious decision to make and should not be treated lightly. Disabled people have fought for decades against prejudice and assumptions about their lives that has, in the past, led to "do not resuscitate" notices being placed on their records. But that is not to deny an individual's right to have an advance directive.

Anyone who proceeds with an advance directive should do so without any pressure or encouragement to proceed. Once such a document is signed it falls within the law described earlier – the Mental Capacity Act, so there is good protection around a directive's authenticity, how and when it was signed and so on.

If you are intent on writing an advance directive and go ahead accordingly, it is important to ensure that your friends and family are aware of its existence so that, if it needs to be invoked, clinicians are shown a copy. Whilst the law with regard to clinicians' adherence to the content of a directive is slightly hazy, it is now generally accepted that a directive falls within common law and that medical staff should abide by an advance directive.

For a more in depth and very helpful discussion of advance directives, visit www.patient.co.uk/showdoc/40025325.

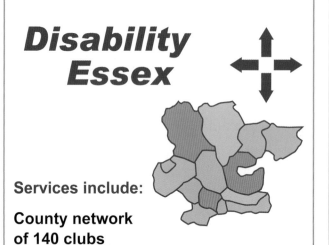
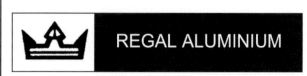
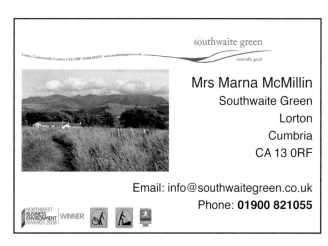

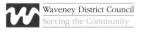

BENEFITS

Many people pay for being disabled in terms of the extra costs involved. For example there can be extra heating costs arising from lack of mobility; you may need to buy equipment, buy more expensive food to meet dietary needs or use taxis rather than public transport or a private car.

While benefits may not meet all these extra costs, they are a legal right for those who meet the entitlement criteria. Make sure you get all you're entitled too. As a general rule, if you are not sure whether you are entitled to a particular benefit, make a claim anyway!

Some benefits are related to a person's extra costs (e.g. Disability Living Allowance), others are specifically for people unable to work (e.g. Employment and Support Allowance), while others are general means-tested benefits designed to top-up income (e.g. Pension Credit). Some benefits overlap, so that if you get one you cannot get another, while others act as a passport (for example receipt of income related Employment and Support Allowance leads to a range of other benefits such as assistance with NHS charges such as prescriptions, vouchers for glasses and hospital travel fares).

There are also some parallel benefit systems for people whose disability resulted from service in the armed forces and industrial injuries.

The benefits system is not only complex but it is frequently changed. The following is no more than an overview.

Disability Living Allowance (Care Component)

People are eligible to apply for the care component of Disability Living Allowance up to the day before their 65th birthday. There is no lower age limit for this component.

Providing the qualifying conditions are met, it may be payable for life. Applicants must have needed help for at least 3 months before claiming and be likely to need it for at least a further 6 months. For children under 16, it would normally be necessary to show that they required more care than would be needed for other children of a similar age.

The DLA is not means-tested or taxable and can be paid in full on top of other benefits.

However social services departments can take it into account when assessing charges for their services.

The DLA Care Component is paid at three levels.

The lower rate is payable to people
who require assistance with their bodily functions from another person for a significant part of the day or who cannot prepare a cooked main meal for themselves. 'Bodily functions' includes hearing, seeing, eating, dressing, bathing, going to the toilet, communicating your needs etc. The cooking test does not apply to children.

The middle rate is payable to people who need either frequent attention or continual supervision throughout the day or prolonged or repeated attention or supervision at night.

The higher rate is for people who need the above level of attention both during the day and at night time. If you are terminally ill you qualify automatically for the higher rate even if you need no care at all when you claim.

An application form for DLA can be obtained from the Benefits Enquiry Line (BEL) on 0800 882200 or from local benefit offices. The former may be preferable as any payment can be backdated to the date that the form was sent out rather than when it was received by the local office.

Attendance Allowance

The Attendance Allowance is a benefit similar to the care component of DLA for people aged over 65. It is payable at two rates depending whether the attention or supervision is required by day or night or by day and night. The assistance must have been needed for 6 months before the benefit can begin to be paid. As with DLA, Attendance Allowance is not taxed or means-tested, can be paid in addition to other benefits and is ignored when assessing other means-tested benefits.

Disability Living Allowance (Mobility Component)

People are eligible to apply for mobility allowance between the ages of 5, or 3 for the higher rate, and 65. The upper cut-off age is important, as no alternative exists for people applying after their 65th birthday. Under-16 year-olds must show that they need substantially more guidance or supervision than a person in normal physical and mental health would require. As with the care component of DLA, applicants must have been eligible for the allowance for three months before their claim and likely to remain eligible for at least six months afterwards.

The mobility component is paid at two levels. The lower rate is for people who are able to walk but cannot do so outdoors without guidance or supervision. This includes people whose mobility difficulties are caused by learning difficulty as well as physical disability.

Conditions such as agoraphobia may also allow someone to obtain the allowance at the lower rate.

The higher rate is for people:

- who cannot walk or are virtually unable to walk;
- who are deafblind
- who have no legs or feet
- for whom walking would lead to a deterioration in their health or a risk to their life
- who have a severe mental impairment and receive the higher rate of the care component

When assessing a "virtual inability to walk" it is the distance, speed and manner of walking without severe discomfort that is taken into account. Environmental factors, say if an applicant lives on a steep hill, are not considered relevant.

Carers Allowance

Carers Allowance is payable to people caring full time for a disabled child or adult who receives the middle or higher rate of DLA or Attendance Allowance. An application can be made while a decision is being made on the payment of DLA. To be eligible for CA the carer needs to meet the following criteria:

- spends at least 35 hours a week caring
- aged between 16 and 65 at the time of your claim
- not in full time education
- not earning more from any employment than the current set amount after allowable expenses are deducted.

CA is not means-tested. However, it is taken into account for other means-tested benefits.

It is taxable and it cannot be paid at the same time as a number of other benefits. However, it does trigger a carers' premium for Income Support and Housing Benefit and provides National Insurance credits and therefore preserves the carer's entitlement to Retirement Pension.

Employment and Support Allowance

Employment and Support Allowance is the new benefit for people whose ability to work is limited by ill-health or disability. It replaces Incapacity Benefit and Income Support paid as a result of incapacity. Over the next few years people receiving those benefits will be moved onto this new benefit.

There are two types of ESA: contributory ESA for those with national insurance contributions and income-related ESA, the means-tested element. Like income support, income-related ESA can help with mortgage interest payments (see Housing section).

During the first 13 weeks of an ESA claim – the 'assessment phase' it is paid at a lower rate. This applies to all new claimants except those who are terminally ill. During this phase you will go through a Work Capability Assessment. This assessment has three elements:

- the limited capability for work test, to see if you should stay on ESA. This is a points-based system which looks at physical and mental health functions. If you get enough points you qualify (if not try claiming Jobseeker's Allowance);

- the limited capability for work-related activity test which is to decide whether you should go into the 'work-related activity' group or the 'support group' (see below) and

❯ the work-focused health assessment (mandatory for those in the work-related activity group or your benefit will be reduced) which collects information about things you can do and assesses what health support, equipment and adaptations would support you back into work.

Those in the work-related activity group are obliged to attend work-focussed interviews with a Personal Adviser to discuss work prospects and draw up an Action Plan outlining activities you could do to help you move closer to or into work. Failure to comply can result in cuts to benefit unless you can show 'good cause' for your failure to attend or participate within a set timeframe.

Those in the support group are not subject to these requirements but they can see a Personal Adviser if they want to.

Certain levels of permitted work are allowed without affecting Employment and Support Allowance:

❯ work for less than 16 hours a week on average, with earnings up to £92.00 a week for 52 weeks;

❯ work for less than 16 hours a week, on average, with earnings up to £92 a week if you are in the Support Group of the main phase of Employment and Support Allowance;

❯ work and earn up to £20 a week, at any time, for as long as you are receiving Employment and Support Allowance;

❯ do Supported Permitted Work and earn up to £92 a week for as long as you are receiving Employment and Support Allowance, provided you continue to satisfy the Supported Permitted Work criteria.

You can claim Employment and Support Allowance by telephone or textphone. An adviser at the contact centre will go though the application with you and fill in the form. You will not have to fill in any forms yourself. Lines are open Monday to Friday, 8 am to 6 pm. Contact centre numbers: ☎ 0800 055 6688. Textphone 0800 023 4888. You can also claim online at www.dwp.gov.uk/eservice

Disability Alliance has produced a detailed guide to ESA available from www.disabilityalliance.org.

All existing IB and new ESA claimants access a programme called Pathways to Work which gives people a tailored package of employment, training and rehabilitation programmes. There is also a Return to Work Credit if you go on to get a job. This is a taxfree payment of £40 per week. It can be payable for up to 52 weeks as long as:

- your job is expected to last at least five weeks

- you are working on average over 16 hours a week

- you are earning no more than £15,000, gross, per year

- you are earning at least the National Minimum Wage

- you have been in receipt of an incapacity benefit for 13 continuous weeks or more.

Working Tax Credit

Working Tax Credit, which incorporates the previous Disabled Persons Tax Credit, is intended to assist people who are in employment or are self-employed but with low incomes. It can be claimed by disabled people who are aged 16 or over and who are working for 16 hours or more a week. It can also be claimed by people who are aged 16 or over and responsible for one or more children and people aged over 25 who usually work at least 30 hours a week.

The amount of credit allowed depends on a means-test and is affected by savings as well as income. It can attract an extra payment as a contribution to paid childcare and is paid at a higher rate for people who:

- are aged 50 or more and have returned to work after receiving out-of-work benefits;
- are in work with a disability which causes a disadvantage in getting a job;
- have a severe disability.

Working Tax Credit and the parallel Child Tax Credit are administered by the Inland Revenue. They are paid along with earnings for people in employment or direct to people who are self-employed.

Child Tax Credit is an allowance for parents and carers of children or young people who are still in full-time education. You may get extra if you care for a disabled child. People receiving Tax Credit should notify the Revenue of changes in their circumstances to avoid over payments that will have to be repaid in the future or to ensure that they are getting all that they are entitled to.

A Helpline for enquiries on Working Tax Credit and Child Tax Credit is available seven days a week on 0845 300 3900. Textphone: 0845 300 3909. Leaflets, also available in Braille, audio and large print, giving further information are available from local HM Revenue & Customs Enquiry Centres or tax offices. Information is also available on www.hmrc.gov.uk/taxcredits

Jobseekers Allowance

Jobseekers Allowance is for people who are unemployed or working less than 16 hours a week and are available for and actively seeking work.

Contribution-based JSA is a flat-rate payment for people with an appropriate National Insurance contribution record who meet a number of other conditions and is payable for up to 6 months. It is taxable.

Income-based Jobseekers Allowance can be paid to people with no or low income and no more than £16,000 in savings. You won't get it if your partner works 24 hours or more a week. It is means tested and taxable. It can top up contribution-based JSA.

Being disabled is a factor in assessing the level of Income-based Jobseekers Allowance.

There are lots of conditions attached to JSA. You will be required to sign a jobseeker's agreement, which contains a description of the type of work you're looking for, the hours you are available and the action you're expected to take to look for work and to improve your job prospects, plus details of any restrictions on your availability for work.

You will have to sign on every fortnight at a Jobcentre Plus office to confirm that you are following your agreement. You will need to attend in-depth interviews with your personal adviser (or your benefit will be stopped, unless you show 'good cause') who can issue a 'jobseeker's direction' requiring you to take a specific step to improve your job prospects.

If you don't comply with one of these directions without 'good cause' your benefit can be stopped for 2 weeks (4 weeks if it's the second time a sanction has been applied). See the Disability Alliance website for further details.

General Benefits

Income Support

Income Support is a means-tested benefit paid to people aged under 60 as a sole benefit or to top-up other benefits. It is only payable to people who are not required to sign on for work such as those who are incapable of work through illness or disability, carers and lone parents.

The amount paid depends on income, savings and family composition. There are supplements, known as premiums, to the basic allowance that are payable in respect of disability, age and carer responsibilities.

If you are claiming Income Support as a result of incapacity now you are likely to be moved onto ESA in the new few years. Existing recipients can continue to claim IS as normal until then. ESA replaces IS paid on grounds of incapacity for new claimants.

Pension Credit

Pension Credit is a benefit that largely replaces Income Support for people aged 60 and above. It is a means tested benefit but the treatment of savings is rather more generous than for Income Support. You get more money if you have caring responsibilities or are severely disabled. Application forms are available by calling 0800 99 1234 or on www.thepensionservice.gov.uk/pensioncredit

Housing Benefit and Council Tax Benefit

Housing Benefit is to help people pay their rent, whether to a local authority, housing association or to a hostel. If you claim Pension Credit, Income Support, Jobseeker's Allowance or Employment and Support Allowance you will automatically be sent a form for this and for Council Tax Benefit. If the person receiving Housing Benefit is out of work and then gets employment, it can be paid for 4 weeks after starting work.

If you are on a low income and rent property or a room from a private landlord you will need to claim **Local Housing Allowance** which is paid straight to you, not the landlord.

Council Tax Benefit is payable in the same way as Housing Benefit to people who are liable for Council Tax, including owner occupiers.

Both of these benefits are administered by local authorities.

Social Fund

The Social Fund is administered by Jobcentre Plus and provides a variety of lump-sum payments, grants and loans in exceptional circumstances. All Social Fund payments are discretionary and for people receiving or eligible for Income Support, income-based Jobseeker's Allowance, income-related Employment and Support Allowance or Pension Credit. They include budgeting and crisis loans, Sure Start Maternity grants and funeral payments.

Of particular relevance to some disabled people will be **Community Care Grants,** which aim to assist people who are moving into their own home from residential or institutional accommodation.

Disability Arising from Employment

The **Industrial Injuries Disablement Benefit** is paid to people who have become disabled as a result of an accident at work or an illness or loss of hearing that has been caused by employment. The amount paid depends on the nature of the disability, the extent to which care is needed and a number of other factors. There are six regional benefit delivery centres which deal with claims for this benefit. This web link will take you to their contact details: http://www.direct.gov.uk/en/ DisabledPeople/FinancialSupport/ OtherBenefitsAndSupport/DG_171827

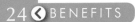

Disability Arising from Service in the Armed Services

A **War Disablement Pension** is payable to people who have become disabled as result of service in the armed forces. The amount depends on the extent of the disability and the total paid is made up of a variety of elements. Payments are handled by the Veterans Agency, which includes the War Pensioners' Welfare Service. Information can be obtained from:

Veterans UK
Norcross, Thornton Cleveleys,
Lancashire FY5 3WP.
Helpline ☎ 0800 169 2277.
Textphone: 0800 169 3458.
@ veterans.help@spva.gsi.gov.uk
Ⓦ www.veterans-uk.info
Advice can also be obtained from service organisations including:

British Limbless Ex-Service Men's Association
185-187 High Road, Chadwell Heath,
Romford RM6 6NA.
☎ 020 8590 1124.
@ headquarters@blesma.org
Ⓦ www.blesma.org

Combat Stress (Ex-Services Mental Welfare Society)
Tyrwhitt House, Oaklawn Road,
Leatherhead KT22 0BX.
☎ 01372 841600.
@ contactus@combatstress.org.uk
Ⓦ www.combatstress.org.uk

Combat Stress provides help and care to ex-Service men and women who have Service related psychological injury through Regional Welfare Officers and treatment centres in Surrey, Shropshire and Ayrshire.

Royal British Legion
199 Borough High Street,
London SE1 1AA.
020 3207 2100.
Ⓦ www.britishlegion.org.uk

The Royal British Legion provides support to those who have served or are serving in the armed forces and their dependants. It fights 36,000 war disablement pension cases and makes around 300,000 welfare visits each year. Telephone information is available on ☎ 0845 7725 725.

Royal British Legion Scotland
New Haig House, Logie Green Road,
Edinburgh EH7 4HR.
☎ 0131 557 2782.
Ⓦ www.rblscotland.org

SSAFA (Soldiers, Sailors, Airmen and Families Association) Forces Help
19 Queen Elizabeth Street,
London SE1 2LP.
☎ 0845 1300 975.
@ info@ssafa.org.uk
Ⓦ www.ssafa.org.uk

Useful Contacts
Benefits Enquiry Line for People with Disabilities
☎ 0800 88 2200.
Textphone: 0800 24 3355.
(8.30am to 6.30pm Monday to Friday and 9am to 1pm on Saturday)

Northern Ireland
☎ 0800 220674,
Textphone: 0800 243787.
(9am to 5pm, Monday to Friday).

The Benefit Enquiry Line (BEL), part of the Department of Work and Pensions, can provide general information and advice on benefits to disabled people, carers and representatives. BEL sends out leaflets and claim packs for a wide range of benefits and also offers a claim form completion service for certain disability related benefits. Braille, large print and taped information is available for some benefits. BEL does not have access to personal records.

Child Poverty Action Group
94 White Lion Street, London N1 9PF.
☎ 020 7837 7979.
@ staff@cpag.org.uk
Ⓦ www.cpag.org.uk

CPAG in Scotland
Unit 9 Ladywell, 94 Duke Street, Glasgow G4 0UW.
☎ 0141 552 3303.

CPAG produces a range of publications including the annual, comprehensive Welfare Benefits & Tax Credits Handbook, which covers means tested and non-means tested benefits and tax credits, and the Paying for Care Handbook. Updated information is given on the website.

Disability Alliance
Universal House, 88-94 Wentworth Street, London E1 7SA.
/Textphone: 020 7247 8776.
@ office.da@dial.pipex.com
Ⓦ www.disabilityalliance.org

The Disability Alliance aims to relieve poverty and improve the living standards of disabled people. It provides information to disabled people, their carers, families and professional advisers on social security benefit entitlement as well as services through publications, factsheets and training courses. It publishes the 'Disability Rights Handbook – A guide to benefits and services for all disabled people, their families, carers and advisers'.

The Family Fund
4 Alpha Court, Monks Cross Drive, York YO32 9WN.
☎ 0845 130 4542 or 0190 462 1115.
Textphone 0190 465 8085.
@ info@familyfund.org.uk
Ⓦ www.familyfund.org.uk

The Family Fund is an independent charity, financed by the governments of England, Northern Ireland, Scotland and Wales, providing grants and information to families with severely disabled or seriously ill children. While operating on a discretionary basis, it works within general guidelines agreed with the Government. The Fund cannot assist with items or help which a local or health authority should be able to provide. Typically the Fund can help with things like holidays, a washing machine or dryer if there is heavy washing as well as grants for clothes or bedding that wears out more quickly through frequent washing. The Fund may also cover play equipment, driving lessons for a main carer and some transport costs if the higher mobility component is not in payment. Application forms can be obtained from the above address or downloaded from the website.

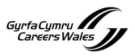
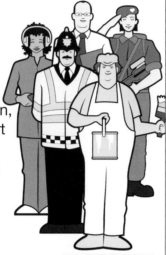

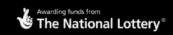

CARERS

The effectiveness of community care often depends on informal networks of care offered by the relatives, friends and neighbours of those who need assistance. In some cases the help given may be only occasional and hardly noticed by the giver, although making a substantial difference to the quality of life of the person being helped. However, in many instances the care is both physically and emotionally demanding.

The importance of the role of carers and their need for support and assistance is becoming better recognised. Under the Carers and Disabled Children Act 2000 people who look after a relative, friend or disabled child and whose caring has a significant impact on their lives can ask the social services to carry out a Carers Assessment. This should be provided regardless of the age of the carer, so would be available for a child assisting an adult or sibling. It can be requested whether or not the person being cared for has had his or her own care needs assessed. It is important to remember that many carers are also disabled people – assessments should recognise this dual identity when relevant.

The law was extended by the Carers (Equal Opportunities) Act 2004 which places a duty on authorities to tell carers of their rights and, when carrying out an assessment, to consider the carer's wishes to work, study or carry out leisure activities. It also gives authorities powers to enlist the help of health, housing and education authorities in providing support for carers.

From April 2007, carers of adults who are in employment have a right under the Work and Families Act 2006 to request flexible working. A booklet 'Flexible Working and Work-Life Balance' that includes information on this new law has been issued by ACAS. This can be obtained by calling 0870 242 9090 or on www.acas.org.uk.

Recent European case law has also established that carers can be discriminated against by association with a disabled person. So, if a carer is, for example, treated badly at work because of the impact of the care they give to a disabled person, a case of discrimination may well exist. Local law centres, citizens advice bureaux and the Equality and Human Rights Commission will be able to advise.

Carers may sometimes be asked to become attorneys, named within a Lasting Power of attorney – see the earlier section on advocacy for more information.

Carers UK
20 Great Dover Street, London SE1 4LX.
☎ 020 7378 4999.
@ info@carersuk.org
Ⓦ www.carersuk.org

Carers Northern Ireland
58 Howard Street, Belfast BT1 6PJ.
☎ 028 9043 9843.
@ info@carersni.org

Carers Scotland
91 Mitchell Street, Glasgow G1 3LN.
☎ 0141 221 9141.
@ info@carersscotland.org

Carers Wales
River House, Ynysbridge Court, Gwaelod y Garth, Cardiff CF15 9SS.
☎ 029 2081 1370.
@ info@carerswales.org

Carers UK works for improved services for carers. It provides advice and information to carers and the professionals who support carers. This is available through its websites, helpline, booklets and factsheets. A network of carers' organisations can provide support. The helpline, CarersLine, is available on 0808 808 7777.

Crossroads – Caring for Carers
10 Regent Place, Rugby CV21 2PN.
☎ 0845 450 0350.
Ⓦ www.crossroads.org.uk

Crossroads NI
7 Regent Street, Newtownards BT23 4AB.
☎ 028 9181 4455.
Ⓦ www.crossroadscare.co.uk

Crossroads Scotland
24 George Square, Glasgow G2 1EG.
☎ 0141 226 3793.
Ⓦ www.crossroads-scotland.co.uk

Crossroads schemes provide services including placing trained carer support workers in the home to take over care tasks to allow the carer a break. There are over 120 Crossroads schemes around the UK. Many schemes provide additional services including young carers' projects, holiday play schemes for disabled children and care for people who are terminally ill.

Princess Royal Trust for Carers
London Office: Unit 14, Bourne Court, Southend Road, Woodford Green, Essex IG8 8HD.
☎ 0844 800 4361.
@ info@carers.org
Ⓦ www.carers.org

Glasgow Office:
Charles Oakley House, 125 West Regent Street, Glasgow G2 2SD.
☎ 0141 221 5066.
@ infoscotland@carers.org

Northern Office:
Suite 6, Oak House, High Street, Chorley PR7 1DW.
☎ 01257 234 070.
@ infochorley@carers.org

Wales Office:
Victoria House, 250 Cowbridge Road East, Canton, Cardiff CF5 1GZ.
☎ 02920 221788.
@ infowales@carers.org

The Princess Royal Trust for Carers supports over 140 Carers' Centres around the country providing information, support and a range of other services. It also provides a website for young carers giving information and support by email and supervised message boards and chat sessions. It is available on www.youngcarers.net

Working Families

1-3 Berry Street, London EC1V 0AA.

☎ 020 7253 7243.

@ office@workingfamilies.org.uk

Ⓦ www.workingfamilies.org.uk

Working Families supports and campaigns for working parents and carers. One of its projects, Waving not Drowning supports parents trying to combine paid work and caring for disabled children. A free newsletter is published for parents and interested professionals and a helpline is available on 020 7253 7243 on Wednesdays, Thursdays and Fridays from 9.30am - 1.00pm and 2.00pm - 4.30pm. For free advice on Tax Credits, flexible working and rights at work parents can call the helpline number 0800 013 0313 which is open Monday to Friday. Make it work for you!, a guidebook for working parents of disabled children gives practical advice on employment rights, benefits and childcare together with stories of how other parents have done it

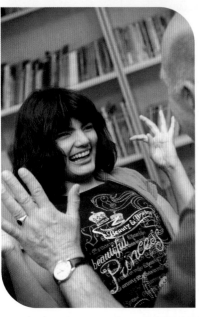
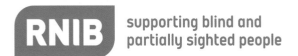
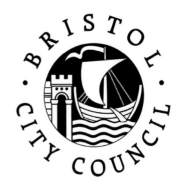
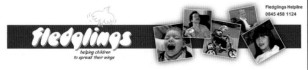
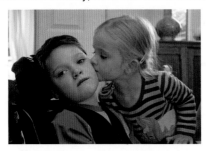

CHILDREN

This section is about the support available to disabled children and their families, focussing on support available before school age and out of school. (See the Education section for details of support available in school.) Disabled children and their families also have important rights and entitlements under benefits legislation community care legislation and housing legislation (see the relevant sections).

If a child is born with, or acquires, an impairment it is critical that parents get as much information as possible about its implications. Not all doctors find it easy to talk openly and honestly to parents about their child's impairment and not all parents find medical terminology easy to understand. Many people, therefore, find they get more positive emotional support and practical information from a parent support group or disability organisation.

With the right support disabled children can grow up to be independent adults with a life as fulfilling and as varied as anyone else. They need to be allowed to take risks and make choices like any other child.

There is a much stronger political focus now on delivering equality and seamless support to disabled children and families.

Children's Commissioners

Every nation of the UK has its own Children's Commissioner responsible for promoting and protecting the rights and welfare of all children and young people (England's Children's Commissioner's remit is weaker: to promote the views and interests of children rather than promote their rights!). They scrutinise and influence policy, can hold inquiries and subpoena witnesses, involve children and young people in their work and provide advice. The England Commissioner can't help with individual cases; the Northern Ireland Commissioner on the other hand can bring or intervene in legal proceedings on behalf of a child.

Children's Commissioner for England
11 Million, 1 London Bridge,
London SE1 9BG.
☎ 0844 800 9113.
@ info.request@11MILLION.org.uk
Ⓦ www.11million.org.uk

Children's Commissioner for Wales
☎ 0808 801 1000.
@ advice@childcomwales.org.uk
Ⓦ www.childcom.org.uk

Northern Ireland Commissioner for Children and Young People
☎ 028 9031 1616.
Minicom 028 9031 6393.
@ listening2U@niccy.org
Ⓦ www.niccy.org

Scotland's Commissioner for Children and Young People
85 Holyrood Road, Edinburgh EH8 8AU.
☎ 0131 558 3733.
Young Person's Freephone
0800 019 1179.
Ⓦ www.sccyp.org.uk

Early Years

Children's Information Services have been established in each Education and Social Services Authority area. An important role is to provide information to parents and others on what is available in the area. Information about appropriate play schools and nursery provision should be available, as should links to LEA services such as home teaching. A CIS may also be the first point of call for information about local parent support groups and assessment and other services offered by voluntary organisations whether locally, regionally or nationally.

Some provide a wider range of information on matters of interest to young people up to school leaving age. The name under which the CIS operates varies from place to place but the contact details should be available from your local authority. They are also listed on a website – www.childcarelink.gov.uk or call 0800 096 0296. In Scotland similar information is available from www.scottishchildcare.gov.uk

Sure Start schemes have been established on a local basis by the Government to further co-ordinate and develop services for children in the areas of greatest need. Although emphasis is given to young children, the remit of Sure Start extends from conception to age 14, or 16 for children with disabilities. Among the services being promoted by Sure Start are Children's Centres, Neighbourhood Nurseries, extended schools and out-ofschool programmes.

In England, Sure Start is being jointly led by the the Department for Children, Schools and Families and the Department for Work & Pensions with a Sure Start Unit that can be contacted on 0870 000 2288 with information on www.surestart.gov.uk
Sure Start programmes also exist in Northern Ireland, Scotland and Wales. In Wales,

Sure Start is part of Cymorth (Children & Youth Support Fund) and administered through Children & Young People's Partnerships that have been established in each local authority.

Early Support is a government initiative, involving the the Department for Children, Schools and Families, the Department of Health and Sure Start to improve services for disabled children aged 0-5. It promotes inter-agency co-ordination, organises training courses for professionals and has published a series of Early Support Information booklets and other material for parents. These are available from voluntary organisations, or can be ordered from DCFS Publications, PO Box 5050, Sherwood Park, Annesley, Nottingham NG15 0DJ or downloaded from or ordered through www.earlysupport.org.uk

Portage

Portage is a home-visiting educational service for pre-school children with special educational needs, which is usually provided by local education authorities. The aim of Portage is to support the development of a young child's play, communication and relationships and give parents the practical help they need to share their child's learning and help with their child's day-to-day learning and activities: www.portage. org.uk

Every Child Matters

Every Child Matters: Change for Children is a an approach to the well-being of children and young people from birth to age 19.

The programme places better outcomes for children firmly at the centre of all policies and approaches involving children's services. These outcomes are:

❯ Be healthy
❯ Stay safe
❯ Enjoy and achieve
❯ Make a positive contribution
❯ Achieve economic well-being

The programme demands that all organisations that provide services to children work together in more integrated and effective ways.

All Children's Trusts are expected to have, by 2010, consistent high quality arrangements to identify all children who need additional help and to intervene early to support them.

A common assessment framework is supposed to be in place in each area already to ensure seamless support.

Extended schools programme

All children should be able to access through schools by 2010:

- A varied range of activities including study support, sport and music clubs, combined with childcare in primary schools
- Parenting and family support
- Swift and easy access to targeted and specialist services
- Community access to facilities including adult and family learning, ICT and sports grounds

For more information:
ⓦ www.everychildmatters.gov.uk

Aiming High for Disabled Children: Better Support for Families

This is a Government programme to: increase the provision of short breaks; enhance families role in shaping services (through Parent Forums); develop more accessible childcare places; give families with disabled children a clear 'core offer' of support they can expect locally; implement a Transition support programme; transform community equipment and wheelchair services and pilot Individual budgets. This is an England programme which involves significant new investment – but the Treasury is making some additional funds available to Wales, Scotland and Northern Ireland too.

Every Disabled Child Matters which campaigns for rights and justice for disabled children has further information: ⓦ **www.edcm.org.uk**

Right to short breaks for disabled children and families

From 2011 in England and Wales local authorities will be under an explicit duty to provide short breaks to disabled children and their families. This is intended to allow children to experience new relationships, environments and positive activities as well as support parents. New funding has been made available to support this. Technically the Chronically Sick and Disabled Persons Act already gives you this right but local authorities have found ways around this. The good thing about the new provision is that it won't just be for crisis situations but to enable parents and carers to maintain and improve the quality of care.

Conductive Education

Conductive Education is a teaching system designed to meet the needs of people with a range of movement disabilities. It teaches people the skills they need to control their bodies and achieve greater independence in their everyday lives. Specially trained Conductors work with the individual to achieve goals that are important to them.

The Foundation for Conductive Education
Cannon Hill House, Russell Road, Moseley, Birmingham B13 8RD.
☎ 0121 449 1569.
@ foundation@conductive-education.org.uk
Ⓦ www.conductive-education.org.uk

The Foundation offers services for people of all ages including:

❯ Free Parent & Child service for up to 3 year olds;
❯ Early intervention service between the ages of 3 and 5 with short-term or continuous service;
❯ Primary school group for 5-11 year olds;
❯ Sessional services for teenagers and children with dyspraxia;
❯ Sessional services for adults with Parkinson's, multiple sclerosis, strokes, head injuries and cerebral palsy and courses for the carers of people with those conditions.

The Foundation offers range of workshops and courses and their website includes a list of other accredited CE Centres.

Schools for Parents, established by Scope, is a network of projects around the country bringing the benefits of Conductive Education to parts of the country without more established Centres. Schools for Parents is for pre-school children with cerebral palsy or other motor learning difficulties, their parents or carers. Parents, in small groups, are taught how to help children learn ways of moving and controlling their bodies so they can eat, walk, dress, communicate and play independently. For more information you can visit Scope's website ⓦ www.scope.org.uk/earlyyears. You can also contact Scope's Early Years Team. ☎ 0808 800 3333. @ response@scope.org.uk

Stays in hospital

If a child has to stay in hospital, the time of visits is usually unrestricted and you may often stay with your child overnight. It is important to talk to one of the nurses about your child's needs so they can be looked after in an appropriate way. The nurses may not be used to nursing children with the particular needs of your child. Your child's social worker will help with organising your visits and dealing with other responsibilities at home whilst your child is in hospital.

Any prolonged or frequent stays in hospital can affect entitlement to benefits.

Child Benefit will be affected if a child is in hospital for over 12 weeks, unless it can be shown that the benefit is used for visits, to buy clothing, etc.

Disability Living Allowance and Carers Allowance are affected after 12 weeks for children under 16; also short stays in hospital will be linked up if they are less than 28 days apart. In addition Carers Allowance will stop if the carer is in hospital for longer than 12 weeks.

Action for Sick Children
36 Jacksons Edge Road, Disley,
Stockport SK12 2JL.
☎ 0800 074 4519
ⓦ www.actionforsickchildren.org

Action for Sick Children has guidelines for the care of sick children before, during and after a stay in hospital in England. It also has information leaflets for parents.

For Scotland and Wales contact:

Action for Sick Children Scotland
22 Laurie Street, Edinburgh EH6 7AB.
☎ 0131 553 6553

AWCH (Wales)
31 Penyrheol Drive, Sketty, Swansea SA2 9JT.
☎ 01792 205227

Association of Children's Hospices

1st Floor, Canningford House,
38 Victoria Street, Bristol BS1 6BY.
☎ 0117 989 7820
Ⓦ www.childhospice.org.uk

ACH represents all UK children's hospice services in Britain together with others that are in the process of establishment. It is concerned with developing best professional practice; improving the provision, regulation and funding of children's hospice services; and promoting the needs of children with life-limiting conditions and their families.

Sick Children's Trust

80 Ashfield Street, London E1 2BJ.
☎ 020 7791 2266.
@ info@sickchildrenstrust.org
Ⓦ www.sickchildrenstrust.org

The Trust provides accommodation for parents and other family members close to major children's hospitals.

Play and Other Equipment

Some toys and play equipment have been designed or have proved useful in the development of disabled children.

Action for Kids

Ability House, 15A Tottenham Lane,
London N8 9DL.
☎ 020 8347 8111.
Textphone: 020 8347 3486.
@ info@actionforkids.org
Ⓦ www.actionforkids.org

Action for Kids offers a national mobility equipment provision service for disabled children and young people and a wheelchair maintenance and repair service. It also offers nationwide family support services including a telephone helpline on ☎ 0845 300 0237 and work related learning services in parts of London and Hertfordshire.

Association of Wheelchair Children

6 Woodman Parade, London E16 2LL.
☎ 0844 544 10 50
Ⓦ www.wheelchairchildren.org.uk

The Association of Wheelchair Children provides specialist wheelchair training, assessments and advice through 1, 2 and 3-day free, mobility skills training courses in all parts of the UK and Ireland for over 500 wheelchair using children and young adults each year.

Fledglings

Wenden Court, Station Approach,
Wendens Ambo, Saffron Walden
CB11 4LB.
☎ 0845 458 1124
@ enquiries@fledglings.org.uk
Ⓦ www.fledglings.org.uk

Fledglings is a not-for-profit organisation established to help parents find specialist equipment, toys and clothing to assist in their children's development. A regular newsletter is issued.

Letterbox Library

71-73 Allen Road, London N16 8RY.
☎ 020 7503 4801.
@ info@letterboxlibrary.com
Ⓦ www.letterboxlibrary.com

Letterbox Library provides children's books by mail order, many of which cannot be obtained elsewhere. Their list includes a diverse and broad-ranging collection of children's disability titles.

MERU

Unit 2 Eclipse Estate, 30 West Hill,
Epsom, Surrey KT19 8JD.
☎ 01372 725203.
Ⓦ www.meru.org.uk

MERU is a charity which designs and custom-makes individual pieces of equipment for children and young people with disabilities, when no ready-made solution exists to meet their needs. It accepts referrals from all over London and the South East of England. MERU also manufactures Bugzi, a powered wheelchair for under-fives, the Moozi low-profile switch joystick, Flexzi – a system for mounting small items and equipment conveniently for the user and Rokzi – add-on accessories that make standard school chairs safer and more comfortable for children with disabilities.

National Association of Toy & Leisure Libraries

68 Churchway, London NW1 1LT.
☎ 020 7255 4600.
@ admin@playmatters.co.uk
Ⓦ www.natll.org.uk

First Floor, Gilmerton Community Centre, 4 Drum Street, Edinburgh EH17 8QG.
☎ 0131 664 2746.

Re-Create Building, Ely Bridge Industrial Estate, Wroughton Place, Cardiff CF5 4AB.
☎ 029 2056 6333.

Toy libraries provide carefully selected toys for families in their local areas to borrow including specialist toys for disabled children. They also usually run play sessions and provide a meeting place for parents and carers. There are over 1000 toy libraries throughout the UK. The NATLL, also known as Play Matters, supports these and promotes the development of new ones. To this end they produce a number of publications, including an annual "Good Toy Guide" which is available via the website.

Sense Toys

13 Barnsbury Terrace, London N1 1JH.
☎ 0845 257 0849.
@ info@sensetoys.com
Ⓦ www.sensetoys.com

Sense Toys is an online shop selling toys and activities and Montessori materials for children with special educational needs. It aims to help stimulate development and language skills through play.

Whizz-Kidz

Elliot House, 10-12 Allington Street, London SW1E 5EH.
☎ 020 7233 6600.
@ info@whizz-kidz.org.uk
Ⓦ www.whizz-kidz.org.uk

Whizz-Kidz aims to improve the quality of life of disabled children in the UK through the provision of customised mobility equipment. It provides help and advice to children and their families and raises awareness of mobility-related issues through national campaigning. It also provides a wide range of specialised mobility equipment not available through the NHS. A network of qualified Mobility Therapists assesses each child for their individual needs. It operates specialist Mobility Centres for children in Birmingham and, in partnership with Disability North, in Newcastle.

Nordoff Robbins

Nordoff Robbins is a national charity (RCN 280960), using the transforming power of music to help disadvantaged people develop creativity, communication skills, confidence and greater wellbeing. Services are provided in schools, hospitals, care homes, private centres and other settings across the UK. For more information visit Ⓦ www.nordoff-robbins.org.uk or ☎ 020 7267 4496.

Companies supplying equipment designed for disabled children include:

Special Needs Toys
5-7 Severnside Business
Park, Severn Road,
Stourport-on-Severn
DY13 9HT.
☎ 01299 827820. Ⓦ
www.specialneedstoys.
com

Winslow
Goyt Side Road,
Chesterfield S40 2PH.
☎ 0845 921 1777. Ⓦ
www.winslow-cat.com

Wise Owl Toys
4 Hardye Arcade,
Dorchester Dorset, DT1
1BZ.
☎ 01305 266 311. Ⓦ
www.wiseowltoys.co.uk

Out-of-School Activities

A local Childrens' Information Service should be able to provide information about the whole range of out-of-school activities that are available in its area. These may include programmes during holidays and mainstream youth organisations, which are increasingly developing integrated services, as well as any special activities such as sports taster days and arts workshops. Some voluntary organisations arrange children's breaks combining activities with peer support and training.

4 Children
City Reach, 5 Greenwich View Place,
E14 9NN.
☎ 020 7512 2112.
@ info@4children.org.uk
Ⓦ www.4children.org.uk

Offers advice and practical support to out-of-school clubs in all stages of development as well as parents, childcare providers, local authorities, employers and Early Years Development and Childcare Partnerships.

Fields in Trust
2d Woodstock Studios, 36 Woodstock
Road, London W12 8LE.
☎ 020 8735 3380.
@ info@fieldsintrust.org
Ⓦ www.npfa.co.uk

Fields in Trust Cymru
Welsh Institute of Sport,
Sophia Gardens, Cardiff CF11 9SW.
☎ 029 2023 0637.

Fields in Trust Scotland
Dewar House, Claverhouse,
Staffa Place, Dundee DD2 3SX.
☎ 01382 817427.

FIT, the trading name of the National Playing Fields Association, works to preserve and encourage the use of outdoor play spaces and playing fields.

Girlguiding UK
17-19 Buckingham Palace Road, London
SW1W 0PT.
☎ 020 7834 6242.
@ chq@girlguiding.org.uk
Ⓦ www.girlguiding.org.uk

Girlguiding UK is the largest organisation for girls and young women and runs Rainbows, Brownies, Guides and Seniors Sections. Its programmes offer a safe female-only space for its members to learn new skills and be involved in community projects both in the UK and overseas. A booklet, Including Disabilities, gives advice to leaders on including people with disabilities in their activities. A network of County Advisors for Members with Disabilities has been established.

Kids

6 Aztec Row, Berners Road,
London N1 OPW.
☎ 020 7359 3073.
Textphone: 020 7359 3520.
@ enquiries@kids.org.uk
Ⓦ www.kids.org.uk

Kids is a national charity providing a range of services for disabled children, their families and siblings. These are organised from regional offices around England and include education for under 5s, family support, information and training, play and leisure. It has particular expertise in promoting inclusive play for disabled children. It is establishing a Young People's Inclusion Network to give disabled young people in England a voice in their inclusion in play and leisure activities.

Scottish Out of School Care Network

Level 2, 100 Wellington Street,
Glasgow G2 6DH.
☎ 0141 564 1284.
@ info@soscn.org
Ⓦ www.soscn.org

SOSCN supports play, care and learning projects for school-aged children in Scotland with a membership drawn from out-of-school care providers, local authorities, voluntary organisations and other bodies. It supports high standards in the over 1000 out-of-school clubs in Scotland. A newsletter and other publications are issued and research carried out.

The Scout Association

Gilwell Park, Bury Road, Chingford,
London E4 7QW.
☎ 0845 300 1818.
Ⓦ www.scoutbase.org.uk

The Scout Association provides activities for all boys including those with disabilities. These activities range from crafts, outdoor pursuits to spiritual development. Its website includes information about activities, events, outings and performances.

Moving On

Connexions

The Connexions service provides integrated advice, guidance and access to personal development for all young people aged 13-19 (up to 25 for young disabled people).

In addition to local services Connexions Direct provides a 7-day a week telephone advice service for young people on ☎ 080 800 13219, Textphone 08000 968 336 or through
Ⓦ www.connexions-direct.com

For other parts of UK contact:
Careers Service Northern Ireland

Lesley Buildings, 61 Fountain Street,
Belfast
☎ 028 9044 1781.
Ⓦ www.careersserviceni.com

Careers Scotland

☎ 0845 8502 502.
Ⓦ www.careers-scotland.org.uk

Careers Wales Association
☎ 0800 100 900.
Ⓦ www.careerswales.com

Transition Information Network

c/o Council for Disabled Children,
8 Wakley Street, London EC1V 7QE.
☎ 020 7843 6006
@ TIN@ncb.org.uk
Ⓦ www.transitioninfonetwork.org.uk

TIN is an alliance of organisations and individuals which aims to improve the experience of disabled young people's transition to adulthood. It is a source of information and good practice for disabled young people, families and professionals. TIN has a magazine and regular email update service but is unable to respond to individual enquiries.

Other Useful Organisations

Brainwave Centre

Huntworth Gate, Bridgwater,
Somerset TA6 6LQ.
☎ 01278 429089.
@ enquiries@brainwave.org.uk
Ⓦ www.brainwave.org.uk

The Brainwave Centre is a charity helping children with physical and cognitive disabilities, whether through brain injury, genetic and chromosome abnormality, or accident. The therapy programme is tailored to the needs of the individual child and parents are taught by the Brainwave therapy team how to carry out the programme in the comfort and familiarity of the home. Regional support workers are available if required. A second centre has been opened in Essex.

British Youth Council

The Mezzanine 2, 2nd Floor,
Downstream Building,
1 London Bridge, London SE1 9BG.
☎ 0845 458 1489.
@ mail@byc.org.uk
Ⓦ www.byc.org.uk

BYC represents and involves young people both individually and as members of youth organisations. It aims to:

❯ Provide a voice for young people;
❯ Promote equality for young people;
❯ Help young people to be more involved in decisions that affect their lives;
❯ Advance young people's participation in society and civic life.

ChildLine

Freepost NATN1111, London E1 6BR.
☎ 0800 1111.
Textphone: 0800 400 222.
Ⓦ www.childline.org.uk

ChildLine offers a free, confidential telephone service for children and young people with any type of problem to speak to a trained volunteer counsellor. It also produces information sheets both for children and adults working with them that can be downloaded from its website and an outreach service, CHIPS, that works with schools.

National Children's Bureau

8 Wakeley Street, London EC1V 7QE.
☎ 020 7843 6000.
Fax: 020 7278 9512.
Ⓦ www.ncb.org.uk

The NCB acts as an umbrella body for voluntary and statutory organisations concerned with children, childcare and family policy in England. It provides information and advice to organisations and policy makers, acts as a focal point for campaigns and issues publications. The National Children's Bureau hosts a number of more specialist bodies including the Council for Disabled Children. Similar bodies in other parts of the UK are:

Children in Northern Ireland

Unit 9, 40 Montgomery Road,
Belfast BT6 9HL.
☎ 028 9040 1290.
Fax: 028 9070 9418.
@ info@ci-ni.org.uk Ⓦ www.ci-ni.org.uk

Children in Scotland

Princes House, 5 Shandwick Place,
Edinburgh EH2 4RG.
☎ 0131 228 8484.
Fax: 0131 228 8585.
@ info@childreninscotland.org.uk
Ⓦ www.childreninscotland.org.uk

Children in Wales

25 Windsor Place, Cardiff CF10 3BZ.
☎ 029 2034 2434.
Fax: 029 2034 3141.
@ info@childreninwales.org.uk
Ⓦ www.childreninwales.org.uk

National Society for the Prevention of Cruelty to Children

Weston House, 42 Curtain Road, London
EC2A 3NH.
☎ 020 7825 2500.
Ⓦ www.nspcc.org.uk

The NSPCC, which operates in England, Wales, Northern Ireland and the Channel Islands, specialises in child protection and the prevention of cruelty to children. It has been protecting children from abuse for over 120 years and has statutory powers to take action in safeguarding children at risk. A free 24 hour Child Protection Helpline is available on (0808 800 5000. Text: 0800 056 0566. E help@nspcc.org.uk

In Scotland contact:

Children 1st

83 Whitehouse Load,
Edinburgh EH9 1AT.
☎ 0131 446 2300.
Ⓦ www.children1st.org.uk

One Parent Families/Gingerbread

255 Kentish Town Road,
London NW5 2LX.
☎ 020 7428 5400.
Ⓦ www.oneparentfamilies.org.uk

One Parent Families has a national project to assist lone parents caring for a disabled child. The Lone Parent Helpline on 0800 018 5026 is open Monday to Friday 9 am - 5pm with extended hours on Wednesdays. The service provides advice and one-to-one help and support on the range of problems facing lone parents who are bringing up children with a disability. In addition lone parents can also get information from the One Parent Families' website and join an on-line forum on its website.

Shared Care Network

Units 63-66 Easton Business Centre,
Bristol BS5 OHE.
☎ 0117 941 5361.
@ shared-care@bristol.ac.uk
Ⓦ www.sharedcarenetwork.org.uk

A charity operating in England, Wales and Northern Ireland promoting short breaks for disabled children with selected families. It co-ordinates over 300 local groups supporting over 10,000 disabled children and their families.
In Scotland contact:

Shared Care Scotland

Unit 7, Dunfermline Business Centre,
Izatt Avenue, Dunfermline KY11 3BZ.
☎ 01383 622462.
Ⓦ www.sharedcarescotland.org.uk

YoungMinds

48-50 St John Street,
London EC1M 4DG.
☎ 020 7336 8445.
Ⓦ www.youngminds.org.uk

YoungMinds is a national charity working to improve the mental health and emotional well-being of children and young people. It has publications and information on its website aimed at children, young people, parents and professionals and operates a Parents Information Service on 0800 018 2138.

DISCRIMINATION

Sometimes people are treated unfairly because of or for a reason relating to their disability. This can be hurtful and distressing but it is against the law. If you experience unfair treatment or if you face barriers to accessing jobs and services, a law called the Disability Discrimination Act (DDA) is there to help you. Disabled people fought hard to get this law on the statute book. It has been improved and added to since 1995 when it was first enacted and gives you:

- A right to fair treatment in recruitment and employment, including a duty on employers to make "reasonable adjustments" to working conditions or the working environment to overcome barriers you face.

- A right of access to goods, services and facilities, including the removal of physical barriers, changes to policies and extra help, where reasonable

- A right of redress against discrimination in the sale and letting of property.

- A right of access to public transport services – buses, trains, stations and airports (plus there are rules about the accessibility of new buses and trains).

- A right not to be discriminated against in education – from nursery education right through to school, college, university and adult learning courses.

An organisation called the Equality and Human Rights Commission is charged with providing advice, information and assistance to disabled people about their DDA rights. It also promotes good practice, undertakes enquiries and has powers to take action against organisations that keep discriminating.

Public sector bodies – like the NHS, local authorities, and Government departments – also have a duty to promote equality for disabled people, including promoting positive attitudes towards disability and encouraging disabled people's participation in all areas of public life.

The Disability Discrimination Act is likely to be replaced by an Equalities Act during 2010, offering similar rights.

Who is protected by the DDA?

The Act protects:-

- People who have, or have had, a disability which makes it substantially difficult for them to carry out normal day-to-day activities. The disability can be physical or sensory, a learning disability, a mental health condition or a long term health problem like diabetes or sickle cell anaemia. It must be long term (have lasted or be expected to last at least a year) or likely to recur.

- People with a history of disability – for example, people who have recovered from a mental illness but continue to experience prejudice.

- People with a severe disfigurement.

- People who are registered/certified blind or partially sighted.

- People with progressive conditions such as cancer, HIV infection or multiple sclerosis (you are covered by the DDA as soon as you have the condition; for other progressive conditions you are covered once your condition begins to have some effect on you).

There is also protection for anyone who is victimised because they helped a disabled person bring a legal case under the DDA. And in employment, people are protected against discrimination and harassment which happens because of an association with a disabled person (e.g. if you are a carer and get treated badly because you have time off to support a disabled child or relative).

The DDA is based on the idea that simply treating disabled people the same as everyone else is not going to deliver real equality; very often disabled people need different or even better treatment to get the same chances and opportunities as everyone else. So the law focuses on positive action to remove barriers, change the way things are done and provide extra support people might need (these are called 'reasonable adjustments'). It also allows disabled people to be treated more favourably than non disabled people - for example if two people are equally well qualified for a job, an employer can decide to employ the disabled candidate.

Education

Disabled people are protected against discrimination in all forms of education and related activities such as meals services, educational trips and student accommodation.

For further information see the Education section of this book.

It is unlawful for general qualifications bodies - bodies which provide general qualifications like GCSEs, A and AS levels, and other non-vocational exams (including Scottish and Welsh equivalents) - to discriminate against disabled people. Exam candidates can expect general qualification bodies to make reasonable adjustments, such as allowing extra time or providing exam materials in alternative formats.

Employment

Part 2 of the DDA outlaws discrimination against disabled people in employment. Employers cannot treat a disabled person less favourably than a non-disabled person when they are recruiting or in terms of people's working conditions (unless they have a 'material and substantial' reason – that's not a get out clause, they have to have a really compelling reason). They also have a duty to make reasonable adjustments for a disabled person so they aren't at a big disadvantage compared to a non disabled person. It does not matter how long you have worked for an employer.

For more information see the Employment chapter of this book.

The DDA also has specific provisions against discrimination in relation to:

❯ occupational pension schemes and insurance obtained through employers (e.g. health insurance);

❯ work experience that someone does as part of their vocational training, e.g. an NVQ in plumbing;

❯ occupations such as police officer, barrister, partnerships and 'office holders' (like judges and members of non-departmental public bodies);

❯ membership of trade organisations (e.g. trade unions);

❯ employment services – such as employment agencies and careers guidance services and

❯ qualifying bodies that make rules about entry into a profession – for example, the Nursing and Midwifery Council.

Local councillors are also covered by the DDA when they are carrying out their official business. But the DDA does not apply to political appointments, local authority cabinet posts or committees.

Goods and Services

Part 3 of the DDA makes it unlawful for the providers of goods, services and facilities to discriminate against a disabled person. Any goods and services that are provided to the general public are covered, regardless of whether you pay for them or who provides them. This includes health, insurance and legal services and retail, sport and leisure facilities.

This means that, unless "justified":

❯ Refusing to serve disabled customers, providing them with inferior services or treating them worse than other customers, is unlawful;

❯ Policies, practices and procedures must be changed (where reasonable) if as they stand, they have the effect of discriminating against a disabled person (for example a restaurant may no longer refuse to admit a person with a guide dog because of a general policy not to admit animals);

❯ Auxiliary aids and services will have to be provided where this is reasonable given the size, resources and nature of the business (this means things like providing information in different formats, giving you extra help);

❯ Where a physical barrier makes it impossible or unreasonably difficult to access a service, the service provider is under an obligation to remove/change it, find a way of avoiding it or provide the service by reasonable alternative means (for example by arranging a meeting at a customer's home rather than in an upstairs office);

A service provider has very limited grounds for 'justifying' discriminatory treatment:

❯ It must be necessary in order not to endanger the health and safety of any person, including the disabled person, or

❯ The disabled person must be incapable of giving informed consent or entering into a legally enforceable agreement (even with accessible information and support);

❯ It is necessary because the provider would otherwise be unable to continue providing the service to members of the public;

❯ A disabled person has been treated less favourably than other people but that was the only way of providing the service to him or her at all;

❯ A disabled person has been charged extra for a service because it's an individually tailored service and the extra cost reflects the higher expense of providing such a bespoke service. (Note: if a service provider is making a reasonable adjustment they cannot charge a disabled person anything for this).

Special rules apply to insurers who are only allowed to charge higher premiums, or to refuse cover, if actuarial or statistical data indicate that the disabled person is at a higher risk.

There is also special provision for guarantees and warranties given by retailers. These usually state that the goods will be replaced if they wear out within a certain period of time and have only been subject to ordinary wear and tear. A retailer may be able to claim justification for not replacing the goods on the basis that as a result of the purchaser's disability the wear and tear was greater than ordinary.

Private clubs with 25 or more members are not allowed to discriminate against disabled members, prospective members or guests and must make reasonable adjustments.

Fair treatment for disabled people in areas like policing and crime prevention, planning and public appointments (these things are called 'public functions' in the legislation) are covered by special provisions too.

Renting or Buying Property

People who sell or let property must ensure that they do not discriminate against disabled people. This covers land and business property as well as residential property. Landlords who let no more than six rooms in their own homes are not affected and nor are those who sell or let their properties privately without advertising.

Landlords cannot refuse to let a flat to you, evict or harass you, offer you a lease on worse terms or stop you using facilities everyone else has access to for a reason relating to your disability. Landlords also have to make reasonable adjustments such as providing tenancy agreements in an accessible format, providing a portable ramp so a wheelchair user can get over a step into their home or waiving a 'no-animals' term in a lease so you can keep an assistance dog. Although they aren't required to change physical features, they do need to consider changing things like signs, doorbells and taps so they are easier to use. If you want to make adaptations to your home, landlords cannot refuse permission unreasonably.

Transport

Access to stations, airports, ticketing services etc is covered by Part 3 of the DDA (see above). The use and provision of transport vehicles such as buses, taxis and trains, trams, minicabs, taxis, car hire and breakdown services is also now covered by Part 3 of the DDA. This means disabled people have protection against less favourable treatment and rights to reasonable adjustments to enable them to use services. Ships and aircraft remain exempt from the DDA Part 3 – although a European law on air transport gives disabled people and people with mobility problems the right not to be refused carriage and the right to certain forms of assistance. The Equality and Human Rights Commission has published a useful guide on "Your rights to fly".

Transport providers are not under duties to overcome physical barriers to vehicles to make them accessible for individual disabled people (except for rental vehicles where they have to look at removing the feature, altering it, providing a way of avoiding it or a different way of making the service available and for breakdown recovery vehicles, where they have to provide an alternative method of making the service available). However, under Part 5 of the DDA, the Government makes accessibility regulations for public service vehicles and rail vehicles. Regulations have been made requiring new built buses, coaches and trains to comply with certain specified accessibility standards, such as width of doors, colour contrasts etc. All buses and coaches must comply with the regulations by 2017 and 2020 respectively. All trains must comply by 2020 at the latest. At the time of writing the Government was consulting on taxi accessibility regulations.

Finally, there are also specific provisions in the DDA preventing licensed taxis and minicabs from refusing to carry or charging more for a disabled person accompanied by a guide or other assistance dog. Drivers can ask to be exempt from this duty on medical grounds.

Challenging discrimination – getting redress

If you are discriminated against by an employer, you can approach the conciliation service ACAS (or its Northern Ireland equivalent) to see if you can resolve the problem without having to go to court. This service is free. Similarly if you are discriminated against in access to goods and services or education, the Equality and Human Rights Commission (in Northern Ireland the equivalent is the Equality Commission) has a free conciliation service you can use.

If you are bringing a legal case under the DDA there are certain time limits you need to be aware of. For employment cases you need to apply to the Employment Tribunal within 3 months of the discrimination taking place; for goods and services cases you need to start a court case within 6 months. There is something called the 'questions procedure' which is useful for getting information you need for your case from employers or service providers.

DDA cases concerning schools must be brought within 6 months. They are heard in the Special Educational Needs and Disability Tribunal and the Special Educational Needs Tribunal in Wales, with similar tribunals in Northern Ireland. Please note though that discrimination cases concerning admission to maintained schools or permanent exclusions are heard by the relevant appeal panels. Scottish schools cases are heard in the Sheriff Court. The unusual thing about schools cases is that, unlike other DDA cases, you cannot get compensation for injury to feelings or financial loss, although schools can be told to give an apology and put things right for you in other ways.

Legal action can be expensive – and there's no legal aid for employment cases, so you could try to get assistance from: your trade union; the EHRC (it can only take on a few cases each year and will have specific criteria); a law centre; the Disability Law Service or your Citizens Advice Bureau.

ACAS

Brandon House, 180 Borough High Street, London SE1 1LW.
☎ 0845 747 4747. Textphone: 0845 606 1600. ⓦ www.acas.org.uk

The Disability Equality Duty

The Government realised it is not fair to expect disabled people to have to challenge discrimination after the event and that public bodies should be doing more to root out discriminatory policies and practices. So a new duty was introduced in 2006 called the "Disability Equality Duty". This means that public authorities (that is local authorities, NHS bodies, Government departments, the police, schools and colleges) must promote equality for disabled people in everything they do.

When they are carrying out their functions (including when they are contracting out services) they must have 'due regard' to the need to: promote equality; eliminate discrimination and harassment; promote positive attitudes towards disabled people; encourage disabled people's participation in public life and take steps to meet disabled people's needs, even if this requires more favourable treatment.

This involves looking at the impact of their policies on disability equality and taking positive action. It's called the 'general duty'.

Certain public bodies have further, specific duties to prepare and implement a Disability Equality Scheme with the involvement of disabled people which must include an action plan against which they can be held to account.

The Duty does not give you extra individual rights. However, if you think a public body is in breach of the general duty you could bring a claim for judicial review of a public authority's action (or inaction) or bring it to the attention of the Equality and Human Rights Commission which has statutory powers to enforce the duty. The EHRC also has powers to ensure public bodies implement their specific duties properly.

Disabled people are using this duty to challenge all kinds of inequalities. For example, disabled people in Harrow used it to stop the local authority restricting social care support. RADAR can provide advice on how you can hold authorities to account under the Disability Equality Duty.

The role of the Equality and Human Rights Commission

The Equality and Human Rights Commission is responsible for promoting equality for disabled people and enforcing the DDA, alongside promoting equality for many other groups. Its role is to:

- help disabled people secure their rights and eliminate discrimination through information, advice and sometimes support with legal cases;

- promote equalisation of opportunities for disabled people with those of non-disabled people;

- promote good practice - working effectively with business and the public and voluntary sectors;

- write the codes of practice and guidance which explain the law in detail;

- undertake enquiries and investigations

- advise Government about how the legislation is working.

It can take enforcement action against organisations that persistently discriminate and is charged with monitoring and enforcing the Disability Equality Duty.

So if you think you have been discriminated against, do contact the EHRC Helpline for advice. For further information contact:

Equality and Human Rights Commission
Arndale House, The Arndale Centre, Manchester M4 3EQ.
☎ 0161 829 8100 (non helpline calls).
@ info@equalityhumanrights.com
Ⓦ www.equalityhumanrights.com

EHRC Helpline England
Freepost RRLL-GHUX-CTRX,
☎ 0845 604 6610. Textphone: 0845 604 6620.

EHRC Helpline Wales
Freepost RRLR-UEYB-UYZL, 3rd Floor, 3 Callaghan Square, Cardiff CF10 5BT.
☎ 0845 604 8810. Textphone: 0845 604 8820.

EHRC Helpline Scotland
Freepost RRLL-GYLB-UJTA, The Optima Building, 58 Robertson Street, Glasgow G2 8DU.
☎ 0845 604 5510. Textphone: 0845 604 5520.

The Disability Discrimination Act relates to the whole of the UK, however in Northern Ireland the role of the EHRC is undertaken by:

Equality Commission for Northern Ireland
Equality House, 7-9 Shaftesbury Square, Belfast BT2 7DP.
☎ 028 9050 0600. Textphone: 028 9050 0589.
@ information@equalityni.org
Ⓦ www.equalityni.org

Other organisations which might be able to help include the Disability Law Service and Law Centres Federation (see the Legal and Consumer Services section for contact details).

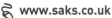

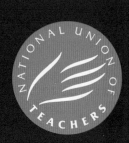

EDUCATION AND SKILLS

Disabled children and young people have the same rights as everyone else to a high quality education, to learn new skills, reach their potential and be fully included in society. Attitudes towards and expectations of disabled children and young people are improving all the time, with more and more youngsters in mainstream education. There's also increasing recognition of the importance of involving disabled children in decisions about their education and learning opportunities.

Key to educational achievement and inclusion is being free from discrimination and getting the practical, tailored support you need to participate in learning on an equal basis. Sometimes it's a struggle for parents and young people to secure this support. This section tells you about how the Disability Discrimination Act can help and what rights disabled children and young people have to get effective support and ensure their educational needs are met. For information on pre-school or early years provision for young children and out-of-school activities see the Children section of this book.

It's never too late to learn. Whatever our age we can all benefit from learning something new for pleasure, learning a new practical skill or boosting our skills for employment. The end of this section provides signposting to sources of advice and information about lifelong learning opportunities.

Discrimination

The Disability Discrimination Act 1995 covers all forms of education: from schools, colleges, universities to adult education providers. The principle behind the legislation is that disabled people should have the same opportunities as non-disabled people in their access to education. Part 4 of the Disability Discrimination Act covers England, Wales and Scotland although, because of the separate educational and legal system, some of the procedures and terminology for England and Wales differ from those in Scotland. Northern Ireland has equivalent legislation.

The Equality and Human Rights Commission has a number of publications on the subject. These include separate leaflets for parents of pupils in schools and one for disabled people in post-16 education. There are also Codes of Practice on the legislation – for schools and for providers of post-16 education and related services. These are invaluable not only in providing information on the legislation but also because they can be quoted and taken into account in any proceedings before a tribunal, appeal panel or court. Its Northern Ireland equivalent is the Equality Commission.

The legislation covers admissions, exclusions and education and related services. The latter not only covers teaching and the curriculum but also services such as educational trips, sports facilities, catering, work experience schemes and student accommodation. (The Disability Discrimination Act also covers schools and colleges as employers and in relation to any non-education services they offer).

The definition of disability under the Disability Discrimination Act is a physical or mental impairment, which has a substantial and long-term affect on a person's ability to perform normal day-to-day activities. This is a lot broader than the definition that exists in the existing law relating to special educational needs.

Under this legislation it is unlawful for a body responsible for an educational establishment to discriminate against disabled pupils or students by

❯ treating them less favourably than others for a reason relating to their disability or

❯ failing to take reasonable steps to avoid putting them at a substantial disadvantage compared with others (reasonable adjustments).

Examples of less favourable treatment would include:

❯ a pupil with a mobility impairment is told she cannot take part in a school trip because of her impairment

❯ a student with dyslexia applies to do a degree in English and is told by a university that it does not accept dyslexic students on its English degree while other students with similar qualifications are offered places on the course

Less favourable treatment can only be justified if it is shown to be for a "material and substantial" reason or is the result of a permitted form of selection.

The duty to make reasonable adjustments is key. It involves changing policies, practices and procedures to enable equal access for disabled pupils and students.

Examples include:-

❯ A school reviews its policies on the administration of medicines and, with assurances that staff are indemnified by the education authority's insurance policy, subsequently allows staff to volunteer to administer medicines;

❯ A school reviews its policy on bullying to ensure that it addresses bullying linked to disability.

What's reasonable depends on things like cost, practicability, health and safety, the maintenance of academic standards, and the impact on other pupils.

An important feature of this element of the law is that it is anticipatory. An educational body cannot just wait to be approached by a disabled pupil or student but must plan for the fact that disabled people will use its services and make proactive improvements in readiness.

For post-16 establishments there are additional requirements to provide additional equipment or staff, referred to as "auxiliary aids and services", that are required by a disabled student. For example:-

❯ A college provides a student with learning difficulties with additional support in her written work so that she can achieve her NVQ qualification

❯ A university arranges for sign language interpretation in lectures for a deaf student

For schools it is assumed that children who require such services will be recognised as having special educational needs and that, therefore, they will be met through the SEN system. However, Local Education Authorities (Education Authorities in Scotland) do have a responsibility to plan improved access to the curriculum and make information available in alternative formats such as Braille and tape.

Colleges and other post-16 establishments are required to make adjustments to the physical features of their premises to avoid discriminating against disabled students. For example a university could install a lift to enable students who are wheelchair users to access lecture rooms on the first floor. Schools have no such duties but they have a duty to plan to increase the accessibility of school buildings.

If a person has been, or thinks they have been, discriminated against the first course of action should be to raise the issue within the organisation; this may be with a head teacher, principal or someone appointed to have responsibility for disability matters. In many instances discrimination may be caused by oversight or lack of awareness that can be quickly rectified. Often there will be an internal system of dealing with complaints if an initial informal approach does not work.

If this does not result in an appropriate reaction the student, pupil or parent can contact the Equality & Human Rights Commission through the EHRC Helpline.

Further action is possible, which has to be initiated within 6 months of the discrimination taking place, or 8 months if the case has gone to the Disability Conciliation Service. This option will vary according to where the alleged discrimination took place, as follows:

- From a school in England and Wales, the Special Educational Needs and Disability Tribunal (SENDIST; SEN Tribunal for Wales) hear most claims of disability discrimination. Separate appeals panels exist to deal with claims of discrimination in relation to admissions and permanent exclusions. If a claim is successful, SENDIST can order the school to carry out any "reasonable" remedy, but not pay financial compensation. Note: Disabled children can't bring DDA cases themselves – their parents have to do it for them.

- From a school in Northern Ireland – the SENDIST hears disability discrimination cases (plus appeals against Education and library Board decisions on special educational needs).

- From a school in Scotland, a claim of disability discrimination can be made by raising an action in the Sheriff Court either by the parent or the child if they are 12 or over. Legal Aid may be available to pay for a solicitor particularly if the child takes the action. Again the Court can order the school to change their policies or practices but cannot impose financial compensation.

- From post-16 education institutions, a claim of discrimination has to be taken as a civil action in a County Court in England, Wales and Northern Ireland, or the Sheriff Court in Scotland. If the case is successful compensation can be awarded as well as an order to stop further discrimination.

Disability Equality Duty

Schools, colleges and universities are subject to the duty to promote disability equality (see the Discrimination section). All (except Scottish Schools) are also subject to the specific duties and should have Disability Equality Schemes and Action Plans.

Equality and Human Rights Commission
See Discrimination section for details.

Special Education Needs and Disability Tribunal (SENDIST)
See listing further in this section.

Special Educational Need

The basic law in England and Wales providing for children with special educational needs is the 1996 Education Act, although this has been significantly amended by the Special Educational Needs and Disability Act 2001. A child with special educational need is one who has a learning difficulty or a disability that makes it harder for them to learn than most children of the same age. A principle of the current legislation is that of inclusion - the majority of pupils with special educational needs will be educated in mainstream schools. Unless his or her parents request it and only in the most exceptional circumstances should a child receive their education in a Special School. The responsibility for assessing whether a child has special educational needs and then of meeting them lies with the Local Educational Authority (LEA).

The process can be started by an approach by the parents or the school or another place of education, such as a nursery. It can take place before the child is of school age as well as at any point within their school career. An early approach is usually recommended. Once an official approach has been made the LEA has up to 6 weeks to make an initial investigation and should also give the parents information on their procedures and give them information on the local Parent Partnership Service and/or organisations providing Independent Parental Supporters.

As a result of the initial investigation, the LEA may decide to carry out a formal assessment of the child's special educational needs. Information about the processes, timescales, etc. and further information on special needs services in the area should be provided to parents together with the contact details of a named LEA officer who will liaise with the parents throughout the process. The assessment will involve the participation of outside professionals such as educational psychologists. Parents should be fully involved in this process including having their own views considered, being kept informed on what is happening and enabled to attend assessments. They can ask for the views of professionals and organisations who know their child to be taken into account. The views of the child should also be given due consideration.

When the formal assessment has been carried out, it may be decided that a formal Statement is prepared. This will include a list of the areas of difficulty in education experienced by the child and all provision that will be made to meet those needs. This "proposed statement" is sent to the parents for further discussion and approval. It is at this stage that a decision has to be made as to the school that the child will attend. Parents will have the opportunity to express their wish between a mainstream or a special school and also, within either sector, their preference for a particular school. Finally, a Statement will be completed containing the name of the school. This should be regularly reviewed and can be altered by agreement to meet changing circumstances.

As an alternative to a Statement a LEA may issue a "Note in Lieu" when the assessment is over. This will explain why a Statement is not considered appropriate, outline the child's special educational needs and make recommendations on how they should be met. All the advice received during the assessment should be attached to the Note in Lieu, which is sent to the parents and, with their consent, to the school.

At all stages in this process there should be the opportunity for parents to challenge decisions that they do not agree with. This may be by direct negotiation, by enlisting the assistance of organisations referred to elsewhere in this book or by using a conciliation or dispute settlement system established by the LEA but containing an independent element. Ultimately parents can appeal against an LEA decision to the Special Educational Needs & Disability Tribunal (SENDIST), an independent body established by the Government. SENDIST publishes guidance for parents considering appealing and operates a Telephone Helpline on special educational need queries.

Special Educational Needs and Disability Tribunal (SENDIST)
Procession House, 55 Ludgate Hill, London EC4M 7JW
☎ SEN Helpline: 0870 241 2555. Discrimination Helpline: 0870 606 5750.
@ sendistqueries@tribunals.gsi.gov.uk Ⓦ www.sendist.gov.uk

SEN Tribunal for Wales
Unit 32, Dole Road Enterprise Park, Llandrindod Wells, Powys LD1 6DF.
Helpline 01597 829800. @ tribunalenquiries@wales.gsi.gov.uk

SENDIST – Northern Ireland
Secretariat, 2nd Floor, Albany House, 73-75 Great Victoria Street, Belfast BT2 7AF.
☎ 028 9032 2894. @ secretary@sentribunal.co.uk

Only a minority of children who at any time have special educational needs will go through all the stages to a formal Statement. Many will have their needs met by teachers adjusting their practices within the classroom – this is referred to as "school action". Others will require the input of extra resources, whether staff or equipment, a process known as "school action plus".

All schools will have a policy on special educational needs and a designated Special Educational Needs Co-ordinator (SENCO). This will normally be a senior member of staff without other school-wide responsibilities; although in small schools it may be the Head or Deputy Head and in large ones there may be a SEN Team. SENCOs' responsibilities will include co-ordinating provision for pupils with special educational needs and overseeing of record keeping on them, liaising with teachers, learning support assistants, parents and external organisations and generally carrying out the school's SEN policy.

The above applies in England and Wales.

Northern Ireland has equivalent legislation – see Ⓦ www.education-support.org.uk for more details. The Education and Library Boards are responsible for meeting special educational needs.

In Scotland the legislation is different and the framework is Additional Support for Learning which gives children with extra support needs similar rights to assessment and support. There is no equivalent yet to SENDIST.

Enquire, The Scottish Advice Service for Additional Support for Learning Princes House, 5 Shandwick Place, Edinburgh EH2 4RG
☎ 0845 123 23 03 (charged at local rates) Textphone: 0131 22 22 439.
Ⓦ www.enquire.org.uk

Enquire publishes The Parent's Guide to Additional Support for Learning.

Further Advice and Information

Parents can obtain information, advice and support from a number of sources during the assessment of their children's needs.

Parent Partnership Services have been established in each Local Education Authority area in England and Wales. These aim to provide parents and carers of children with special educational needs with information, advice and guidance so that they can make informed decisions on their children's education. They will frequently provide an initial point of contact outside the school for parents who are concerned that their children have or may have special educational need. They should be able to introduce parents who want one to an Independent Parental Supporter if this is required and have information on voluntary organisations, self-help groups and other organisations that may be appropriate both locally and nationally.

The **National Parent Partnership Network,** established by the Council for Disabled Children with funding from the Department for Education and Skills, provides a forum for local services to share learning, experience and information. The NPPW website includes the contact addresses for Parent Partnership Services throughout England – **www.parentpartnership.org.uk**

Advisory Centre for Education

1c Aberdeen Studios, 22 Highbury Grove, London N5 2DQ.
☎ 020 7704 3370.
@ enquiries@ace-ed.org.uk
Ⓦ www.ace-ed.org.uk

ACE works for an education system that supports all children and promotes the active involvement of parents in their children's education. Their work is based on the provision of information, advice and support to parents who have problems with their children's schooling. This is usually given by telephone, although disabled people unable to use a phone can use the internet. A wide range of publications is available, as is training for education professionals and local advisors. An advice line is open on ☎ 0808 800 5793 Monday-Friday 10am-5pm.

The Alliance for Inclusive Education

336 Brixton Road, London SW9 7AA.
☎ 020 7737 6030.
@ info@allfie.org.uk
Ⓦ www.allfie.org.uk

This is a network of local groups and individuals working for a fully inclusive education system. Publications include Snapshots of Possibility highlighting examples of inclusion.

Centre for Studies on Inclusive Education

New Redland Building, Frenchay Campus, Coldharbour Lane, Bristol BS16 1QU.
☎ 0117 328 4007.
@ admin@csie.org.uk
Ⓦ www.csie.org.uk

The CSIE produces publications and organises seminars and training on issues relating to inclusive education. They publish the Index for Inclusion for early years and schools to help break down educational barriers.

Disability Equality in Education

Unit GL, Leroy House, 436 Essex Road, London N1 3QP.
☎ 020 7359 2855.
@ info@diseed.org.uk
Ⓦ www.diseed.org.uk

Disability Equality in Education is a charity providing training and resources to education bodies promoting the full inclusion of disabled people in the education system.

Enquire

Children in Scotland, 5 Shandwick Place, Edinburgh EH2 4RG.
☎ 0131 222 2425.
Textphone: 0131 222 2439.
@ info@enquire.org.uk
Ⓦ www.enquire.org.uk

Enquire is the Scottish advice service on Additional Support for Learning, funded by the Scottish Government and managed by Children in Scotland. It is available to children and young people with additional support needs, their parents and carers and to professionals working with them.
A telephone Helpline is available on ☎ 0845 123 2303.

The Good Schools Guide collates public information on a wide range of schools with the comments submitted by parents   and other independent, interested people. A number of schools catering for children with special needs are highlighted including some ainstream schools that "do well by" pupils with special needs. The Guide is expanding the coverage of such schools and welcomes help in identifying them.

For further information contact Good Schools Guide, 3 Craven Mews, London SW11 5PW
☎ 020 7801 0191.
Ⓦ www.goodschoolsguide.co.uk

inclusion.ngfl.gov.uk – a website that is part of the National Grid for Learning that includes a catalogue of resources to support individual learning needs and news, information and advice on inclusion issues.

Independent Panel for Special Education Advice
6 Carlow Mews, Woodbridge, Suffolk IP12 1EA.
☎ 01394 446575. Ⓦ www.ipsea.org.uk
Advice Line: 0800 0184016

IPSEA provides free independent advice and support in England and Wales to help ensure that the views of parents/carers and children are taken fully into account when children's needs are assessed and decisions made about special educational provision and school placement. This can include providing second professional opinions and representation at a Special Educational Needs Tribunal, often by a volunteer who has been helped by IPSEA in the past. Booklets giving guidance for parents and others are available.

National Association of Independent Schools and Non-Maintained Special Schools (NASS)
PO Box 705, York YO30 6WW.
☎ 01904 624446.
Ⓦ www.nasschools.org.uk

NASS represents the interests of independent special schools and seeks to promote high standards and appropriate practices. The association was set up in 1997 for voluntary organisations and now also admits private special schools as associate members. A list of member schools is included on the NASS website.

Network 81
1-7 Woodfield Terrace, Stansted, Essex CM24 8AJ.
☎ 0845 077 4056. Helpline: 0845 077 4055.
Ⓦ info@network81.org
Ⓦ www.network81.org

A national network of parents working for properly resourced inclusive education for children with special educational needs. Network 81 offers support and information through a telephone Helpline, publications, training, information days and a network of befrienders and supporters.

Parents for Inclusion
Unit 1, Winchester House, Kennington Park Business Centre, Cranmer Road, London SW9 6EJ.
☎ 020 7735 7735,
Free Helpline: 0800 652 3145.
@ info@parentsforinclusion.org
Ⓦ www.parentsforinclusion.org

A parent based organisation working for an inclusive education system with appropriate resources. They provide support for parents through their Helpline and by representation and also offer a wider training and consultancy service on inclusive education.

The following organisations are among those that have developed educational computer software and other resources to help pupils with special educational needs:

Don Johnston Ltd
18/19 Clarendon Court,
Calver Road,
Winwick Quay,
Warrington WA2 8QP.
☎ 01925 256500.
Ⓦ www.donjohnston.co.uk

Inclusive Technology Ltd
Riverside Court,
Huddersfield Road,
Delph,
Oldham OL3 5FZ.
☎ 01457 819790.
Ⓦ www.inclusive.co.uk

LDA
Pintail Close, Victoria Business Park,
Nottingham NG4 2SG.
☎ 0845 120 4776.
Ⓦ www.ldalearning.com

Logotron Software/REM Ltd
Great Western House,
Langport TA10   9YU.
☎ 01458 254700.
Ⓦ www.logo.com, www.r-e-m.co.uk

SEMERC
Angel House, Sherston,
Malmesbury SN16 0LH.
☎ 01666 843200.
Ⓦ www.semerc.com

Sherston Publishing Ltd
Angel House, Sherston, Malmesbury
SN16 0LH.
☎ 01666 843200.
Ⓦ www.sherston.com

Making the transition from school to Further Education

Further education is a great way to learn new skills and broaden your career options. A big range of academic and vocational courses are available.

If you had a statement of special educational needs while at school, you should have a 'transition plan' giving details of the support you'll need once you leave. Most transition plans start to get drawn up in Year 9. You should get a letter from your headteacher inviting you and your parents to a review meeting where the plan should get drawn up. You can also have an advocate for this meeting. Plans are meant to be holistic – they are about what you want to achieve in the next few years and what support you will need to live as independently as possible. They should cover every aspect of your life, including education, employment, housing, health, transport and leisure activities. Think beforehand about the things you want to study, what you want to do when you leave school and what support you think you will need.

After the meeting you should get a copy of the Transition Plan and a copy will go to your headteacher and other relevant professionals. The education department of your local authority is responsible for making sure that you receive all the support and services that are listed as necessary for you in your Transition Plan. You should have another review meeting each school year to update your Transition Plan.

If you stay on at school to attend sixth form, you'll continue to get the help set out in your statement. Your sixth form or college should pay for your learning support.

Before you start college visit it so you can see what's available and talk the Learning Support Adviser or Special Education Needs Co-ordinator.

Colleges are expected to make provision for disabled students such as additional teaching for dyslexic students, an interpreter for deaf students, materials in alternative formats, and specialist computer software.

Learning and Skills Council

Cheylesmore House, Quinton Road, Coventry CV1 2WT.
☎ 0845 019 4170. @ info@lsc.gov.uk Ⓦ www.lsc.gov.uk

The Learning and Skills Council is responsible for all post-16 education and training, except universities. It works with Further Education and Sixth Form Colleges, training organisations, Jobcentre Plus and representatives of community groups. In addition to the national office in Coventry, there are 9 regional offices and a network of local partnerships across England delivering a range of locally determined activities. Information on these is given on the website. Changes to this organisation are coming in from 2010

Its arrangements for funding Colleges include an element for improving the physical accessibility of premises for disabled students.

Weymouth College, after three external audits, has put together a Disability Equality Plan which has been incorporated in the overall College Improvement Plan and which has led to a number of initiatives. An inclusion brochure has been produced and is available to all students and parents. A Disability Forum has been started to give students and staff a place to discuss issues and receive information on the progress of action points. Improvements have been made to the accessibility of the College website and premises and a Student Liaison Officer has been appointed to encourage further student participation.

A number of specialist colleges and other establishments offer further education courses for disabled students whose needs are not met by local provision. Young people with complex disabilities or severe learning difficulties may be assessed as needing further education up to the age of 25. Specialist colleges generally operate on a residential basis and include training in life skills along with other vocational and academic courses. There may be close liaison with mainstream colleges in the area or a positive aim of providing a stepping-stone to other training or education possibilities. Information on specialist colleges can be obtained from:

Association of National Specialist Colleges (NATSPEC)
☎ 0117 973 2830. Ⓦ www.natspec.org.uk

NATSPEC represents specialist further education establishments with the aim of promoting opportunities for education and training, in residential or day settings, for students with disabilities and learning difficulties. A list of full and associate members is available on the organisation's website.

Higher Education

Many disabled students go on to higher education and undertake courses at Universities. As with further education colleges these will have an officer or department charged with advising and co-ordinating services for disabled students and prospective students.

Disabled Students' Allowances help with costs incurred as a direct result of a disability in attending a higher education course. It will depend on an individual's requirements and may include the cost of specialist equipment, non-medical helpers and travel. The DSA is not means tested and does not have to be repaid. It is available for full time study on both undergraduate and postgraduate courses and to both full and part-time students, although the latter must be studying at least half time. Bridging the Gap: a guide to the disabled students' allowances in higher education is issued annually by the Department for Business, Innovation and Skills and can be down loaded from www.direct.gov.uk

DSAs are for students living in England and Wales but broadly similar systems exist in Northern Ireland and Scotland. In most cases applications have to be made to:

❥ **Student Finance England** ☎ 0845 300 50 90; textphone 0845 604 44 34 (for those starting courses in 2009-2010, otherwise apply to your local authority

❥ in Wales – your local authority – information is available at www.studentfinancewales.co.uk

❯ the **Education & Libraries Board** in Northern Ireland
- www.studentfinanceni.co.uk

❯ the **Student Awards Agency for Scotland** in Scotland - www.saas.gov.uk.

Access and assessment centres around the country provide specialist information on the equipment and support that students with disabilities will need to study at university or college. These carry out an assessment of course related need for prospective students or current students who become disabled. This will be carried out by an independent assessor with knowledge of the range of equipment and educational strategies that may be suitable. LEAs and other agencies will use these assessments when making decisions on DSAs, as will other funding bodies. An assessment may also be useful when planning study strategies with the college or university or in obtaining equipment beyond that covered by a DSA.

'Is University for You? A Guide for Deaf Students' – encourages prospective students to think about going to university and includes information on how to apply, the communication and financial support available and exam arrangements. The Guide is available on video, DVD or CD Rom and can be ordered from RNID Information Line, 19-23 Featherstone Street, London EC1Y 8SL. ☎ 0808 808 0123. Textphone: 0808 808 9000. E information@rnid.org.uk

Skill
Unit 3, Floor 3, Radisson Court,
219 Long Lane, London SE1 4PR.
☎/Textphone: 020 7450 0620.
@ skill@skill.org.uk
Ⓦ www.skill.org.uk

Skill Northern Ireland
Unit 2, Jennymount Court,
North Derby Street, Belfast BT15 3HN.
☎/Textphone: 028 9028 7000.
@ admin@skillni.org.uk
Ⓦ www.skillni.org.uk

Skill Scotland
Norton Park, 57 Albion Road,
Edinburgh EH7 5QY.
☎/Textphone: 0131 475 2348.
@ admin@skillscotland.org.uk

Skill Wales/Sgil Cymru,
Suite 14, 2nd Floor, The Executive
Centre, Temple Court, Cathedral Road,
Cardiff CF11 9HA.
☎ 029 2078 6506.
@ temp@skillwales.org.uk

Skill, the National Bureau for Students with Disabilities, gives information and advice to disabled students on how to maximise their experiences in education, volunteering, training and entry to employment. Skill publishes Into Higher Education annually giving information on making applications, obtaining support, grants and benefits and also a list of higher education institutions and their Disability Co-ordinators. The list is also available on the website.

Lifelong learning

If you are not sure where to begin, there's lots of free, impartial advice about learning, careers and courses from services like Careers Advice and nextstep. It will be able to tell you about your options and funding you could get to help pay towards your learning. You can meet a trained adviser face-to-face, have a conversation over the phone or contact an adviser by email. Contact Careers Advice free on 0800 100 900 or visit http://careersadvice.direct.gov.uk.

Apprenticeships provide career training for those who have finished full-term education, and enable them to develop skills and gain qualifications while in employment. National Apprenticeships helpline: 0800 015 0600. W ww.apprenticeships.org.uk

The Get On helpline provides confidential advice to adult learners who wish to improve their literacy, numeracy or language skills. ☎ 0800 66 0800 (freephone) W http://geton.direct.gov.uk. Opening Hours 8.00 am to 10.00 pm, seven days a week.

Distance and Home Learning

To be able to study from home has many advantages for some disabled people particularly as the benefits of improved technology become more widely available. Distance learning has moved on from simply being correspondence courses.

Open & Distance Learning Quality Council

16 Park Crescent, London W1B 1AH.
☎ 020 7612 7090.
@ info@odlqc.org.uk
Ⓦ www.odlqc.org.uk

The ODL QC is an independent body that operates a registration scheme for providers of home study, distance and online learning and other open learning courses. To register providers have to meet certain standards, which are then monitored. If anything goes wrong with a course from an accredited provider ODL QC can help sort out the problem. Most accredited organisations are concerned with professional and vocational qualifications but some work with school-age learners and others provide more general or academic courses.

National Extension College

Michael Young Centre, Purbeck Road, Cambridge CB2 8HN.
☎ 01223 400200.
@ info@nec.ac.uk Ⓦ www.nec.ac.uk

The National Extension College is a charity that has helped people of all ages fit learning into their lives for over 40 years. They support 20,000 people a year on over 100 home study courses. Their Carers' into Education Project, in the Midlands and Eastern England, is specifically for those who need to fit studies around caring responsibilities.

Open College of the Arts

Michael Young Arts Centre, Redbrook Business Park, Wilthorpe Road, Barnsley S75 1JN.

☎ 0800 731 2116.

@ enquiries@oca-uk.com

Ⓦ www.oca-uk.com

The OCA is an open-access college offering home-study courses on painting, drawing, textiles, photography, music, writing and design. No formal qualifications are required and there are no age limits. The tutors are all practising artists, photographers, composers, writers or designers.

The Open University

Walton Hall, Milton Keynes MK7 6AA.

☎ 01908 274066.

Ⓦ www.open.ac.uk

Since its foundation the Open University has welcomed disabled students and developed its services for them. It now has more disabled students than the entire student numbers at some universities. A wide range of advice and guidance for Open University students with a disability is available online and in the leaflet Open to your needs which summarises the support services and facilities that are available to prospective students. Drawing on its experience, advice about teaching inclusively for staff in higher education is available on www. open.ac.uk/inclusiveteaching/

Other Useful Contacts

ACE Centre Advisory Trust

92 Windmill Road, Headington, Oxford OX3 7DR.

☎ 01865 759800.

@ info@ace-centre.org.uk

Ⓦ www.ace-centre.org.uk

The ACE (Aiding Communication in Education) Centre provides a focus on information and expertise in the use of technology as an aid to communication. The organisation provides an assessment service, which sets out clear and realistic recommendations for an individual's special needs to improve their physical and communication difficulties. It offers training to teachers, therapists, parents and enablers to ensure that technology is used appropriately with the people they support. The ACE Centre serves the southern part of England and Wales.

For similar services in the north contact:

The ACE Centre North

Hollinwood Business Centre, Albert Street, Hollinwood, Oldham OL8 3QL.

☎ 0161 684 2333.

@ enquiries@ace-north.org.uk

Ⓦ www.ace-north.org.uk

In Scotland contact:

The CALL Centre (Communication Aids for Language and Learning)

University of Edinburgh, Paterson's Land, Holyrood Road, Edinburgh EH8 8AQ.

☎ 0131 651 6235/6236.

@ info@callcentrescotland.org.uk

Ⓦ callcentre.education.ed.ac.uk

British Educational Communications and Technology Agency (Becta)

Milburn Hill Road, Science Park, Coventry CV4 7JJ.

☎ 024 7641 6994.

@ becta@becta.org.uk

Ⓦ www.becta.org.uk

Becta, is the Government's partner in developing and delivering an information and communications technology strategy to schools and other education and training establishments providing a link between ICT and education.

ContinYou

Unit C1, Grovelands Court, Grovelands Estate, Longford Road, Exhall, Coventry CV7 9NE.

☎ 024 7658 8440.
@ info.coventry@continyou.org.uk
Ⓦ www.continyou.org.uk

London, 31-33 Bondway, Vauxhall, London SW8 1SJ

☎ 020 7587 5080.
@ info.london@continyou.org.uk

Anchor Court, Keen Road, Cardiff CF24 5JW.

☎ 029 2047 8929.
@ info.cardiff@continyou.org.uk

Loughborough Innovation Centre, Loughborough University, Epinal Way, Loughborough LE11 3EH.

☎ 01509 222417

ContinYou provides a range of programmes to encourage people of all ages to take up learning opportunities. They seek to establish links between education, health and employment particularly for people who have gained the least from formal education and training.

LearnDirect

PO Box 900, Leicester, LE1 6ER.

☎ 0800 101 901.
Ⓦ www.learndirect.co.uk

LearnDirect provides courses in computers, skills for life, management and languages through local learning centres in England and Wales and online.

The Makaton Charity

Manor House, 46 London Road, Blackwater, Camberley, Surrey GU17 0AA.

☎ 01276 606760.
@ info@makaton.org
Ⓦ www.makaton.org

Makaton is a language programme of signs, symbols and speech. It has been developed for children with severe communication and learning disabilities to encourage communication, language and literacy skills. Often it serves as a voice to communicate with family members, teachers, friends and others. The Makaton Charity provides a wide range of resources (books, videos, training packs, etc.) for parents, carers and professionals. A network of qualified, licensed Tutors provides training on a regional and local basis for people wishing to learn Makaton and how teach it to people with learning difficulties.

nasen

nasen House, 4/5 Amber Business Village, Amber Close, Amington, Tamworth B77 4RP.

☎ 01827 311500.
@ welcome@nasen.org.uk
Ⓦ www.nasen.org.uk

nasen, formerly the National Association for Special Educational Needs, aims to promote the education and training of all those with special educational needs and provide a forum for those working in the field. It has around 6000 members in 60 branches around the country. A wide range of publications is issued including the regular journals Support for Learning and British Journal of Special Education. Other activities include conferences, courses and exhibitions.

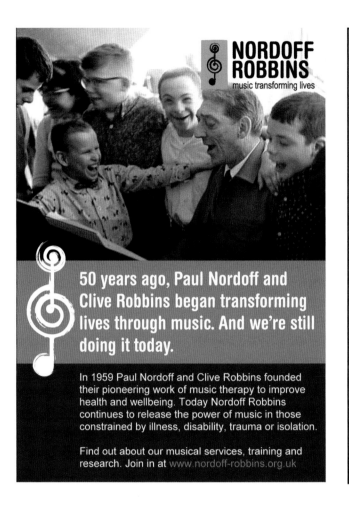
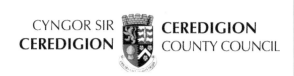

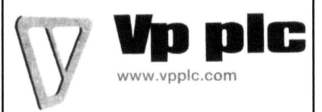
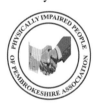

OAASIS

Freepost RLYY-TAUC-YRYS,
1-2 Brock House, Grigg Lane,
Brockenhurst SO42 7RE.

☎ 0800 9020732. Ⓦ www.oaasis.co.uk

OAASIS aims to give impartial advice and information to parents and teachers of children with special educational needs. It is part of Cambrian Education Services, a provider of independent special schools and colleges.

Scottish Sensory Centre

Moray House, University of Edinburgh, Holyrood Road, Edinburgh EH8 8AQ.

☎ 0131 651 6501.
Textphone: 0131 651 6067.
Ⓦ www.ssc.education.ed.ac.uk

The SSC promotes and supports new and effective practices in the education of children and young people with sensory impairments. It organizes short courses and produces a regular newsletter and other publications and videos. Bibliographies and resource documents are available online. A postal lending service gives access to specialist collections of books, videos and other material.

SEBDA

Room 211, The Triangle, Exchange Square, Manchester M4 3TR.

☎ 0161 240 2418.
@ admin@sebda.org Ⓦ www.sebda.org

SEBDA (Social, Emotional and Behavioural Difficulties Association) provides its members, who are teachers and others working with or for children and young people who are said to have 'BESD', who are disaffected with behavioural difficulties or who have mental health difficulties with up-to-date information, support and professional development through its magazine/ newsletter, research journal, networking and web-site.

EQUIPMENT

Everyone uses pieces of equipment to make their lives easier or more convenient – from TV remote controls to a long handled shoehorn. The right piece of equipment can make daily life easier for disabled people and bring greater freedom and control. These can vary from the extremely simple, such as a pick-up stick or an extended tap turner, to the highly sophisticated, such as an environmental control system.

Many items can be provided by local authorities or through the health service. For local authority provision of equipment, contact your social worker or occupational therapist. For health service items, including wheelchairs, walking aids or communication aids contact your GP. Throughout England there are now Community Equipment Services bringing together the social services and health provisions, with the exception of wheelchairs. Equipment may also be supplied in relation to education and employment (see the relevant sections).

Equipment can also be bought privately. However, it is advisable to seek advice and try the equipment out before you buy. This is particularly important if the equipment is expensive and/or complicated.

British Healthcare Trades Association

New Loom House, Suite 4.06, Back Church Lane, London E1 1LU.
☎ 020 7702 2141.
@ bhta@bhta.net
Ⓦ www.bhta.net

The BHTA represents manufacturers and suppliers of a wide range of equipment for disabled people. Members have signed up to a stringent Code of Practice (which has achieved stage one of the Office of Fair Trading (OFT) Consumer Codes Approval Scheme) and an arbitration service is available in the event of any dispute. BHTA Registered Persons are committed to a personal Code of Conduct as well.

Social Services Departments can provide advice as part of their assessment of a person needs and more generally through their community OT service. For example Durham County Council operates a number of centres giving advice and also where some equipment is available for sale.

Some equipment is eligible for zero-rating for VAT when supplied for the personal use of a disabled person's. The supplier should know about this and information is given in VAT Notice 701/7 from HM Revenue and Customs.

Disabled/Independent Living Centres offer impartial advice on equipment for disabled people to individuals, families, carers and professionals. All centres have a range of products and information on display and many centres also run various training days, produce leaflets and provide other services. Information on Centres throughout the UK is available from Assist UK, Redbank House, 4 St Chad's Street, Manchester M8 8QA. ☎ 0870 770 2866. Textphone: 0870 770 5813. @ general.info@assist-uk.org W www.assist-uk.org

To find the opening hours, range of services or to make an appointment at your nearest Disabled Living Centre call:

Bargoed - Centre for Help & Advice for the Disabled
☎ 01443 822262

Beckenham – BATH Independent Living Centre
☎ 020 8663 3345

Bexley - Inspire Community Trust
☎ 01322 341638

Birmingham – Assist Centre for Independent Living.
☎ 0121 464 4942.
Textphone: 0121 464 7565

Boston - Disabled Living Centre
☎ 01205 367597

Brighton & Hove - Daily Living Centre
☎ 01273 296132/3. Textphone: 01273 725421

Bristol - Living
☎/Textphone: 0117 965 3651

Bury St Edmunds - West Suffolk Disability Resource Centre
☎ 01284 748888. Textphone: 01284 748881

Castleford - Ability Centre
☎ 01977 724012

Croyden – Independent Living Centre
☎ 020 8664 8860

Dewsbury - Social Services Information Point
☎/Textphone 01924 325070

Doncaster - South Yorkshire Centre for Independent Living
☎ 01302 892949. Textphone: 01302 892968

Dudley – Assisted Living Centre.
☎ 01384 813695

Dundee – Independent Living Centre & Community Equipment Centre
☎ 01382 307635

Dunstable - Disability Resource Centre
☎ 01582 470900

Durham – Home Independence Service
☎ 0191 386 0742

Eastbourne – East Sussex Disability Association
☎ 01323 514515. Textphone: 01323 514 502

Edinburgh - Lothian Disabled Living Centre
☎/Textphone: 0131 537 9190

Elgin - Moray Resource Centre
☎ 01343 551339. Textphone: 01343 551376

Exeter – Independent Living Centre
☎ 01392 687276

Gainsborough – BRC Disabled Living Centre
☎ 01427 816500

Grangemouth – Dundas Resource Centre
☎ 01324 504311

Halton – Independent Living Centre
☎ 01928 563340

Hillingdon - Independent Living Centre
☎ 020 8848 8260.
Textphone: 020 8848 8323

Leeds – William Merritt Disabled Living Centre and Mobility Service
☎/Textphone: 0113 305 5332

Leicester - BRC Disabled Living Centre
☎ 0845 373 0217.
Textphone: 0116 262 9465

Lincoln - Disabled Living Centre
☎ 01522 545111

Liverpool - Disabled Living Centre
☎ 0151 296 7742.
Textphone: 0151 296 7748

London – Disabled Living Foundation
☎ 0845 130 9177.
Textphone: 020 7432 8009

Lowestoft - Waveney Centre for Independent Living
☎/Textphone: 01502 405454

Mablethorpe – BRC Disabled Living Centre
☎ 01507 478574

Manchester – Regional Disabled Living Centre
☎ 0161 214 5959

Middlesbrough - Independent Living Centre
☎ 01642 250749

Milton Keynes - Centre for Integrated Living
☎ 01908 231344.
Textphone: 01908 231505

Newcastle Upon Tyne – Disability North
☎ 0191 284 0480.

Newton Aycliffe – Home Independence Service
☎ 01325 327467

Northwich - Independent Living Centre
☎ 01606 79260

Nottingham - Disabilities Living Centre
☎ 0115 985 5780

Oxford - Dialability
☎ 08456 251 251

Paisley - Hospital Discharge Team
☎ 0141 847 4959

Papworth Everard – Cambridgeshire Independent Living Centre
☎ 01480 830495

Semington - Wiltshire & Bath Independent Living Centre
☎ 0845 111 0079

Shipley - Disability Equipment Bradford
☎ 01274 589162

Shrewsbury - Independent Living Partnership
☎ 01743 210820

Southampton – Equipment Demonstration & Advisory Service
☎ 023 8071 8855

Stamford – Disability Living Centre
☎ 01780 480599

Swindon – Independent Living Centre
☎ 01793 643966

Truro - Cornwall Mobility Centre
☎ 01872 254920

Warrington - Centre for Independent Living
☎ 01925 240064

Welwyn Garden City – Hertfordshire Action on Disability
☎ 01707 384260.
Textphone: 01707 324581

Wilmslow – East Cheshire Independent Living
☎ 01625 374080

www.livingmadeeasy.org.uk is a free and impartial website, developed by the Disabled Living Foundation (DLF) that aims to provide advice and information on daily living equipment available in the UK and other aspects of independent living.

Exhibitions

Exhibitions of equipment for disabled people can be a good way of finding out what is available. Although some of these attract visitors from across the country or even abroad, others have a more local catchment area or deal with specific types of equipment. In most cases the exhibitors include disability organisations as well as equipment manufacturers and suppliers. News of events that are coming up is given in local newspapers, disability media and at local or regional information points. Among the largest regular exhibitions are:

Mobility Roadshow
Mobility Choice, Crowthorne House, Nine Mile Ride, Wokingham, Berkshire RG40 3GA.
☎ 0845 241 0390.
Ⓦ www.mobilityroadshow.co.uk

Since 1983, the annual Mobility Roadshow has provided a showcase of a wide range of mobility products and services. It offers the opportunity to test drive a wide variety of adapted cars and specialist conversions, including drive-from-wheelchair options, plus other hands-on driving, sports and leisure activities, as well the chance to meet companies and organisations specialising in mobility and independent living. The 2009 show takes place at Kemble Airfield near Cirencester from 4th-6th June.

NAIDEX & Kidequip – in Birmingham (NEC) in the Spring

DNEX – in the Autumn in Newcastle

Remap
D9 Chaucer Business Park, Kemsing, Sevenoaks, Kent TN15 6YU.
☎ 0845 130 0456.
Ⓦ www.remap.org.uk

Although the range and sophistication of equipment is ever increasing, there are still occasions where nothing exists to meet a particular requirement of a disabled person. Remap panels consist of volunteer engineers and other professionals who make specific pieces of equipment, which are not available commercially. There are around 100

Remap panels located throughout the UK.

Foundation for Assistive Technology

31 Scarborough Street, London E1 8DR.
☎ 020 7264 8955. @ info@fastuk.org
Ⓦ www.fastuk.org

FAST works to promote useful research and development on equipment or assistive technology for disabled people. It brings together current or prospective users of assistive technology with researchers, developers, manufacturers and other service providers to become partners in the design, development and assessment of new products.

Ricability

30 Angel Gate, City Road,
London EC1V 2PT.
☎ 020 7427 2460.
Textphone: 020 7427 2469.
@ mail@ricability.org.uk
Ⓦ www.ricability.org.uk

Ricability is an independent research charity publishing practical and unbiased consumer guides for older and disabled people on a range of products and services. Recent reports have covered childcare products for disabled parents, household products, the use of public transport by wheelchair users, driving and car adaptations, community alarms and telecommunications equipment and services. All guides are on the Ricability website and most are available in Braille, tape and large print. A publications list and ordering details can be obtained from the address above.

Homecraft Rolyan

Nunn Brook Road, Huthwaite, Sutton in Ashfield, Notts NG17 2HU.
☎ 08444 124 330.
Ⓦ www.homecraft-rolyan.com

Homecraft Rolyan, a long established

company, supplies a wide range of equipment for disabled people of all ages and the elderly. All products are available on its website or in a catalogue that can be ordered from the address above.

Keep Able

Unit 3-4 Sterling Park, Pedmore Road, Brierley Hill DY5 1TB.
☎ 0844 8881337.
@ homeshopping@keepable.co.uk
Ⓦ www.keepable.co.uk

Keep Able supplies products which aid independent living. They can be ordered by post or over the internet. A list of retail stores across the UK is available on its website.

Nottingham Rehab Supplies

Clinitron House, Excelsior Road, Ashby-de-la-Zouch LE65 1JG.
☎ 0845 120 4522.
@ customerservice@nrs-uk.co.uk
Ⓦ www.nrs-uk.co.uk

NRS stocks a range of over 2000 products for elderly and disabled people and those in rehabilitation.

Promedics ADL Ltd/Able2

Moorgate Street, Blackburn BB2 4DP.
☎ 01254 619000.
@ enquiries@able2.eu
Ⓦ www.able2.eu

Promedics ADL's Able to Care catalogue includes a wide range of items to assist daily living available through the website or by mail order.

Totally Active

The Enterprise Centre, Duke Close, West Way, Andover SP10 5AP.
☎ 0800 138076.
@ info@totallyactive.co.uk
Ⓦ www.totallyactive.co.uk

Totally Active, part of the Simplyhealth

Group, can supply independent living and mobility equipment. Free brochures are available on its website.

Hiring equipment on a short or medium term basis may be a useful option in some circumstances. Some local suppliers offer this service. Those operating on a national basis include:

Direct Mobility Hire Ltd

Warren House, 201A Bury Street, Edmonton, London N9 9JE.
☎ 0800 0929322.
@ info@directmobility.co.uk
Ⓦ www.directmobility.co.uk

Direct Mobility hires and sells a wide range of mobility, bath, toilet and bed equipment. Next day delivery possible in the area around London.

The Great British Mobility Group Ltd

5A & 6A The Grange Business Park, The Grange, Hewish BS24 6RR.
☎ 0800 980 0978.
@ sales@greatbritishmobility.com
Ⓦ www.greatbritishmobility.com

This company has adjustable beds and chairs, bath lifts, hoists and scooters for hire. It can deliver with 48 hrs notice. A free brochure can be ordered on its website.

Theraposture Ltd

Kingdom Avenue, Northacre Industrial Park, Westbury BA13 4WE.
☎ 0800 834654.
@ info@theraposture.co.uk
Ⓦ www.theraposture.co.uk

Theraposture provides a wide range of adjustable beds, chairs and other equipment. This company offers short term rental programme for adjustable beds (2 weeks rental minimum).

Clothing & Footwear

People who have limited dexterity or restricted movement may have difficulty putting on or fastening clothing. Some disabled people have problems finding off-the-peg clothes that fit properly or that there can be above average wear and tear on particular areas of clothing.

Often these problems can be overcome by selecting clothes that are easy to use or by altering them at home but sometimes you may need to get clothes specially made or bought by mail order from specialist suppliers. Some stores offer a shopping assistance service that can be useful for disabled people.

Comfortable, correctly fitting footwear is important. If an impairment causes shoes to wear unevenly, it may be advisable to buy shoes that can easily be repaired. A doctor or consultant can refer people who need built-up or orthopaedic shoes or boots to a specialist fitter. Many people, however, find that they are most comfortable in sandals or trainers or choosing shoes with easy fittings. A chiropodist or physiotherapist should be able to give advice on appropriate footwear.

Able 2 Wear

53 Donaldson Street, Kirkintilloch,
East Dunbartonshire G66 1XG.
☎ 0141 775 3738.
@ info@able2wear.co.uk
Ⓦ www.able2wear.co.uk

Privately owned company that designs
and manufactures all types of clothing
for wheelchair users and others who
have difficulty buying clothes that fit
them.

British Footwear Association

3 Burystead Place,
Wellingborough NN8 1AH.
@ info@britfoot.com
Ⓦ www.britfoot.com

BFA is a trade association representing
British footwear manufacturers and
British based footwear brands.

Cosyfeet

The Tanyard, Leigh Road, Street,
Somerset BA16 0HR.
☎ 01458 447275.
@ comfort@cosyfeet.co.uk
Ⓦ www.cosyfeet.com

Cosyfeet supply a wide range of extra
wide-fitting footwear that is suitable
for people with very wide, swollen or
bandaged feet. It also stocks a range of
other products for lower body comfort
and foot and leg care. As well as shoes
the items covered include socks, hosiery,
slippers and foot creams. These can be
ordered from its website, catalogue or
through its own and other outlets.

Disabled Living Foundation

380-384 Harrow Road, London W9 2HU.
☎ 020 7289 6111.
Textphone: 020 7432 8009
@ info@dlf.org.uk Ⓦ www.dlf.org.uk

Among DLF's many information sheets
on daily living and mobility equipment,

which can be obtained from the above
address or download from the website,
are the following on clothing and
footwear:

❯ Choosing a bra

❯ Clothing for continence and
incontinence

❯ Clothing for people with sensitive skin

❯ Clothing ideas for people who rip
clothing

❯ Clothing ideas for wheelchair users

❯ Dressing for warmth

❯ Equipment to assist with dressing
& putting on footwear

❯ Finding suitable footwear

❯ Specialist clothing services.

Seenin

Aydon South Farm, Aydon, Corbridge,
NE45 5PL.
☎ 01434 634457.
@ info@seenin.co.uk
Ⓦ www.seenindesign.co.uk

Suppliers of protective wear, including
bibs, kerchiefs, overalls and wheelchair
covers, for disabled children and
adults. Seenin can also provide bespoke
garments.

Communications

There is a wide range of equipment available to help people communicate ranging from 'simple' adaptations to keyboards and voice-activated mobile telephones for visually impaired people to speech replacement devices. Advances in technology have given disabled people new opportunities to improve their communication. Some items may be supplied through the health service, possibly from a Communication Aids Centre, or be prescribed by a hospital consultant. In appropriate circumstances equipment can be supplied for use in education or employment. Other equipment may be supplied by a charity or will have to be bought privately.

Augmentative and alternative communication (AAC) is a general term used to describe methods of communication used to supplement speech and/or writing when these are impaired and includes unaided systems such as signing and gesture, as well as aided techniques ranging from picture charts to the most sophisticated computer technology currently available. Because communication is a two-way process, AAC techniques can be used to enhance both the understanding of speech as well as the individual's ability to express him/herself.

AbilityNet

Acre House, 11/15 William Road,
London NW1 3ER.
☎ 0800 269545.
@ enquiries@abilitynet.org.uk
Ⓦ www.abilitynet.org.uk

AbilityNet, a national charity, is the UK's leading provider of advice on computing and disability. It provides a freephone advice and information line, individual assessments, a wide range of factsheets and awareness training for professionals.

Aidis Trust

3 Gunthorpe Street, London E1 7RQ.
☎ 020 7426 2130.
@ info@aidis.org
Ⓦ www.aidis.org

The Trust helps disabled people communicate more easily and effectively through the use of technology. It offers advice, assessment, installation and ongoing training and support. It runs a programme of workshops and can supply selected equipment through its website.

BT Inclusive Communications

81 Newgate Street, London EC1A 7AJ.
☎ 0800 800 150.
Textphone: 18001 0800 800 150.
Ⓦ www.btplc.com/inclusion

BT offers a number of services and products to assist people who have problems with communications. These are listed on its website and in BT's Communications Solutions Guide. This is available free by calling the above number.

Communication Matters

ACE Centre, 92 Windmill Road,
Headington, Oxford OX3 7DR.
☎ 0845 456 8211.
@ admin@communicationmatters.org.uk
Ⓦ www.communicationmatters.org.uk

Communication Matters, also known
as ISAAC UK, is a national charity
focusing on the needs of people who
have complex communication needs
who may benefit from using some
form of augmentative and alternative
communication (AAC) system. Members
include those involved in the AAC field
either personally or professionally. A wide
range of publications are available on
or can be ordered through its website.
The Communication Matters National
Symposium, regional study days and
equipment road shows are organised
throughout the year.

ITCH Network

British Computer Society, Block D,
North Star House, North Star Avenue,
Swindon SN2 1FA.
@ info@itcanhelp.org.uk
Ⓦ www.itcanhelp.org.uk

The ITCH (IT Can Help) Network, part of
BCS, uses skilled volunteers to assist
disabled people with computer problems
in their own homes, at other venues
or remotely. It works in partnership
with AbilityNet (see above) and disabled
people needing assistance should
contact the AbilityNet Client Helpline
0800 269545 or E enquiries@abilitynet.
org.uk

1 Voice - Communicating Together

PO Box 559, Halifax HX1 2XT.
☎ 0845 330 7862.
@ info@1voice.info
Ⓦ www.1voice.info

1 Voice provides a network of information
and support for people who use a
communication aid to act as their voice
as well as for their families and carers.
It provides opportunities for personal
contact in a variety of settings and also
through the internet.

Ricability

30 Angel Gate, City Road,
London EC1V 2PT.
☎ 020 7427 2460.
Textphone: 020 7427 2469.
@ mail@ricability.org.uk
Ⓦ www.ricability.org.uk

Ricability, an independent research
charity, has been commissioned by the
Government to carry out tests on the
ease of use of digital TV products. The
research is detailed and unbiased and
reports are now available on over 130
products, including digital televisions,
indoor aerials, set top boxes and digital
TV recorders. There is also information
on its website about going digital,
including details of the Help Scheme to
provide assistance for some older and
disabled people in the lead up to the
digital television switchover.

RNID Typetalk

John Wood House, Glacier Building,
Harrington Road, Liverpool L3 4DF.
☎ 0800 7311 888.
Textphone: 18001 0800 500 888.
@ helpline@rnid-typetalk.org.uk
Ⓦ www.typetalk.org

Typetalk is the national telephone relay
service whereby people with a speech
or hearing impairment who use a
textphone can communicate with those
using standard telephones. The service
operates on a 24-hour basis throughout
the year.

RNID Solutions is a catalogue of products specifically chosen to help solve everyday problems for deaf and hard of hearing people. It contains over 200 products. Contact RNID Products Customer Services on ☎ 01733 361199, Textphone 01733 238020, Fax 01733 361161 or order a copy online at www.rnid.org.uk/shop

The Sequal Trust

3 Ploughman's Corner, Wharf Road, Ellesmere, Shropshire SW12 0EJ.
☎ 01691 624222.
@ info@thesequaltrust.org.uk
Ⓦ www.thesequaltrust.org.uk

The Sequal Trust raises funds to provide communication aids and adaptations for people with speech/movement disabilities and/or learning difficulties. These aids are provided on loan basis for as long as the need exists.

UCanDoIT

Highfield House, 4 Woodfall Street, London SW3 4DJ.
☎/Textphone: 020 7730 7766.
@ info@ucandoit.org.uk
Ⓦ www.ucandoit.org.uk

UCanDoIT is a charity that teaches computer and internet skills to blind, deaf, and disabled people on a one-to-one basis at home. Students are taught how to e-mail, surf the web, and access news groups and chat rooms.

The basic course consists of 10 lessons – each lesson costing from just £5, and lasting between one and two hours. All the tutors are vetted by the police and have extensive IT backgrounds. Students have been aged from 12 to 80. Being taught one-to-one at home has many advantages, in particular, immediate answers to questions and no need to face the trek to sometimes intimidating large colleges. The course and the material can be geared to an individual's needs. Initially operating in Greater London, there are now trainers in Edinburgh, Glasgow, Devon, Wales, Cheshire, Kent, Merseyside, Sussex and Milton Keynes with a remote training project under way.

Vodafone Disability Services

Vodafone House, The Connection, Newbury RG14 2FN.
☎ 08700 733222.
Textphone 020 8288 8038.
@ disability.access@vodafone.co.uk
Ⓦ www.vodafone.co.uk/Disabilityservices

Vodafone Disability services offer help and advice to make phones and services more accessible and easier to use to the elderly and people with disabilities. A wide range of services for disabled customers are outlined in various guides and booklets. These are available as downloads on its website or copies can be ordered online.

See the Education Section for information on organisations concerned with the provision of communications equipment for disabled children and young people at school.

Equipment for blind and partially sighted people

Thousands of accessible and inclusive products such as talking, tactile and easy-to-see watches, telephones, kitchen equipment, and mobility aids are available from RNIB. www.onlineshop/rnib.org.uk. For more information telephone Customer Services on 0845 702 3153 / 01733 37 53 50 or email cservices@rnib.org.uk. RNIB also has a grants programme for equipment.

RNIB Talking Book Service offers over 15,500 audio books, paid for by annual subscription and delivered through the post to your door. Subscription gives you access to a variety of ways to choose your books including support from professional librarians. Talking Books are in the Daisy format which lets you skip to a new chapter or insert a bookmark using a lightweight player with accessible controls. To join Talking Books contact RNIB Helpline on 0303 123 9999 or email helpline@rnib.org.uk. The full loan annual subscription, which includes the loan of a player, costs £76. The books only annual subscription costs £50

Mobility Equipment

The NHS provides free, long-term loan of a manual wheelchair to a person with a permanent mobility need. Powered indoor/outdoor wheelchairs may be provided if a person is assessed that they cannot propel a manual one. An occupational therapist or physiotherapist at home will carry out an assessment, in hospital or at the local NHS wheelchair service. This should also include the need for accessories such as cushion, armrests and trays. In some areas people may be offered a voucher towards the cost of a privately purchased wheelchair if the assessment shows that they would benefit from features not available on models provided by the NHS.

Most powered outdoor chairs and sports models have to be bought privately, and as with all equipment, advice should be sought from a Disability Living Centre.

Get Mobile is a free RADAR guide to buying a scooter or powered wheelchair, giving information on the types of products available, assessing needs, methods of purchase, funding, operating costs and other matters.

People with the higher rate of the mobility component of DLA can consider using the **Motability Powered Wheelchair & Scooter** scheme to lease or buy a powered buggy or wheelchair on hire purchase over one to four years. For information call 0845 607 6260

Class 3 powered wheelchairs and scooters, those capable of speeds of up to 8mph and that are not restricted to footpaths, must be registered for road use, licensed in the exempt 'disabled' taxation class and display a nil duty vehicle licence (tax disk). Class 2 scooters are exempt. Owners of mobility scooters who fail to register their vehicles may face fines. The DVLA says that in order to first register and license a class 3 "invalid carriage", the user needs to complete form V55/5 (for used vehicles) or V55/4 (for new vehicles) - and take or send it to their nearest DVLA local office. Evidence of the vehicle's age needs to be submitted with the application together with documentation confirming the keeper's name and address. The number at the DVLA to get the forms and local office addresses is 0870 243 0444, the website is www.dvla.gov.uk.

You can get walking aids such as crutches, walking sticks and frames (if you have a medial need for them) on loan from a local hospital or community equipment service.

Local Red Cross branches operate a short term medical equipment loan service for wheelchairs, other mobility aids and some other equipment. Contact details are in local phone books or can be obtained from:

British Red Cross
44 Moorfields, London EC2Y 9AL.
☎ 0844 871 1111. @ information@redcross.org.uk
Ⓦ www.redcross.org.uk

A similar service may be available from local disability organisations and some equipment suppliers also offer a hire service.

Environmental Control Systems

Environmental control systems enable people to operate a wide range of equipment and appliances within their home from a single control. They can be provided through the NHS after an assessment by a medical consultant who acts as the environmental control assessor for the area. An occupational therapist would be involved in the installation and the individual design of the functioning of the system. The equipment is provided on loan and is maintained and serviced without charge.

Assistance Dogs

There is a long tradition of trained guide dogs assisting blind people in their mobility. In recent years dogs have been trained to help a wider range of disabled people. The following organisations are members of Assistance Dogs UK:

Canine Partners

Mill Lane, Heyshott, Midhurst, West Sussex GU29 0ED.
☎ 0845 658 0480.
@ info@caninepartners.co.uk
Ⓦ www.caninepartners.co.uk

Dogs for the Disabled

The Frances Hay Centre, Blacklocks Hill, Banbury Oxon OX17 2BS.
☎ 01295 252600.
@ info@dogsforthedisabled.org
Ⓦ www.dogsforthedisabled.org

The Guide Dogs for the Blind Association Burghfield Common, Reading RG7 3YG.
☎ 0118 983 5555.
@ guidedogs@guidedogs.org.uk
Ⓦ www.guidedogs.org.uk

Hearing Dogs for Deaf People

The Grange, Wycombe Road, Saunderton, Princes Risborough HP27 9NS.
☎/Textphone: 01844 348100.
@ info@hearingdogs.org.uk
Ⓦ www.hearingdogs.org.uk

Hearing Dogs for Deaf People is a UK charity that selects and trains dogs, mostly from rescue centres or similar backgrounds, to alert deaf people to important sounds and danger signals at home, the workplace or public buildings. Hearing dogs provide their deaf partners with greater independence, confidence and security.

Support Dogs

21 Jessops Riverside, Brightside Lane, Sheffield S9 2RX.
☎ 0114 261 7800.
@ supportdogs@btconnect.com
Ⓦ www.support-dogs.org.uk

In addition to training dogs to assist physically disabled people, Support Dogs trains seizure alert dogs to support people with epilepsy and some other conditions.

> Dog Assistance in Disability provides dog training for disabled people enabling them to train their pets in general obedience and specialised tasks to help in daily life. Contact Dog AID Headquarters, 43 Sir Alfreds Way, Sutton Coldfield, West Midlands B76 1ET. Ⓦ www.dogaid.org.uk

Telecare

The aim of telecare is to enable people to live independently while providing access to help when needed and reassurance. Telecare services range from pendant alarms through to more complex sensor arrangements.

Most parts of the country are covered by a telecare pendant alarm service from a local or national organisation.

In recent years, local authorities, housing associations and third sector organisations have been putting into place telecare sensor services. Generally, a base unit will plug into a wall telephone socket and a nearby electrical socket. Sensors are placed around the home that will send alerts to the base unit then down the telephone line to a control centre where a response will be provided. For example, a flood detector would pick up water on the floor of a bathroom or kitchen and send a message through the base unit to the control centre. A computer screen in the control centre provides information about the address and location of the detector and arrangements for calling the user or a carer, family member, response service or emergency services. The control centre staff are generally able to maintain communication with the user during the emergency to provide reassurance. Telecare services can provide information about the best sensors to use in the home to handle different situations including smoke, temperature, movement and inactivity, falls and epileptic seizures.

Telecare services are often called careline, linkline, helpline, community alarm or given a local name associated with the organisation providing the service.

A small number of local authorities and health trusts have been testing telehealth systems that can monitor respiratory and heart conditions at home - these services are very limited at this time. These services include regular home monitoring of blood pressure, blood sugar, weight and other vital signs. If these measurements are outside of certain levels, healthcare professionals (e.g. specialist nurses, community matrons) are alerted and will take appropriate follow up action.

"Calling for Help – a Guide to Community Alarms" produced by the independent research charity Ricability, gives consumer information on the various community alarm systems and the points to consider when choosing between them. Single print copies can be obtained by sending an A4 addressed envelope with 56p in stamps to Ricability, 30 Angel Gate, City Road, London EC1V 2PT. ☎ 020 7427 2460. Textphone: 020 7427 2469. Ⓦ www.ricability.org.uk

Schemes can be run by local authorities, voluntary organisations and commercially and may be provided on a local basis or over a wider, even national area. Similarly the level of charges and charging procedures vary. However, the social services department may be able to assist with the cost for someone assessed as needing this service. Equipment costing under £1,000 should be provided free.

Information on local services can be obtained from local authorities and other local information points.

Telecare Services Association
Suite 8 Wilmslow House, Grove Way, Wilmslow, Cheshire SK9 5AG.
☎ 01625 520320. @ admin@telecare.org.uk
Ⓦ www.telecare.org.uk

TSA represents organisations running, funding and providing equipment for community alarm or telecare services. Its members conform to a code of good practice. Information about services around the country can be given by phone or obtained from its website.

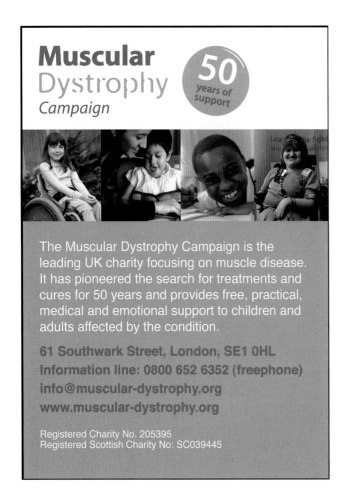
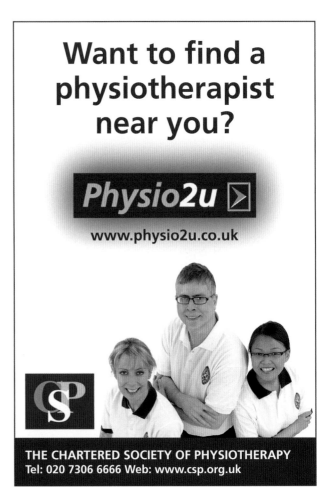
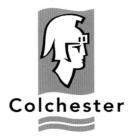

HEALTH SERVICES

As disabled people we often need to use health services just like everyone else – for everything from flu to advice on quitting smoking. We also may need to use the health service for our impairment – for instance, we may use a spinal injury unit or need radio-therapy for cancer (which is classified as a disability under the DDA).

Health services specifically for our impairment should increasingly offer us choice and control. If we have 'continuing care' needs we may be entitled to an individual budget – so we can know how much is allocated to our needs and can (if we wish) manage our own supports and services using that money.

More detailed information on the arrangements for treatment and support for conditions associated with our impairments can be obtained from specialist organisations on, for instance, spinal injury, cancer and the like.

The rest of this section concentrates on using health services just like everyone else.

Crucially, health service providers have responsibilities as both employers and service providers under the Disability Discrimination Acts. So, for example, if you need, for impairment related reasons, any (or all or more) of the following, you have a right to ask for it and for it to be delivered without question:

❯ Large print information about medicines, surgical intervention, treatments and so on

❯ A longer appointment time to help you fully understand what's under discussion

❯ Fully accessible premises to be seen or treated within

❯ Equal treatment – for example, as much access to regular screening services as anyone else

The GP is the first point of contact for community health services, most of which are provided on a GP's recommendation, and for referral to hospital. Home visits can be arranged if you are unable to get to the surgery. You can register with any

GP who will accept you and can change GP without giving a reason. A list of GPs in the area can be obtained from the Primary Care Trust (PCT) for your area. The PCT is also responsible for allocating patients to GPs if you have difficulties in finding one or if you have been refused entry to a GP list or been removed from a list.

NHS Direct
☎ Helpline 0845 4647. Textphone: 0845 606 4647.
Ⓦ www.nhsdirect.nhs.uk

NHS Direct is a 24-hour nurse-led advice and information service in England and Wales providing information on:

❯ What to do if you or a member of your family is feeling ill;

❯ Particular health conditions;

❯ Local healthcare services including doctors, dentists and late opening pharmacies;

❯ Self-help and support organisations.

In Scotland contact NHS24 on
☎ 0845 424 2424. Ⓦ www.nhs24.com

In Wales see
Ⓦ www.wales.nhs.uk

In Northern Ireland see
Ⓦ www.hscni.net

An increasing number of NHS Walk-In Centres provide a face-to-face service similar to NHS Direct.

A GP can refer patients to a health visitor or community nurse. Health visitors are specialist nurses employed to give advice and assistance on family and infant health and associated issues. Community nurses visit people at home to give nursing care, such as changing dressings, and to assist with the provision of home nursing equipment.

General information on the organisation of health services is provided in Your Guide to the NHS available from surgeries and other information points or from the Department of Health Publications, PO Box 777, London SE1 6XH. Information can also be found on Ⓦ www.direct.gov.uk

Help with costs

Some aspects of health care which are normally charged for, such as prescriptions (see a more in depth discussion later in this section) and sight or dental examinations, are available free for certain groups of people including children, those over 60, people with certain medical conditions, pregnant women, people with a War Disablement Pension and people receiving income related benefits. Other people on low incomes, including those waiting for a benefit claim to be settled, can claim under the NHS Low Income Scheme by filling in form HC1 available from a Social Security office or hospital.

Chiropody

Chiropody, sometimes also called podiatry, concerns the care of the feet. This is far more than cosmetic, and for people with conditions such as diabetes it is frequently essential. Elderly people can find their mobility enhanced by chiropody treatment, as do people with foot deformities. Disabled people, children, pregnant women and pensioners are entitled to free chiropody treatment under the NHS. Most chiropodists/podiatrists will treat people at home if they are unable to get to a clinic. Treatment can be obtained by self-referral or by referral from a GP or health visitor.

The Society of Chiropodists & Podiatrists
1 Fellmonger's Path, Tower Bridge Road, London SE1 3LY.
☎ 020 7234 8620.
Ⓦ www.feetforlife.org

The professional body for chiropodists and podiatrists can advise on locating the society's members. Its website also gives information on foot care.

Continence

Many people are understandably embarrassed about discussing problems they may be having with incontinence, although it may help to know that such problems are very common. It has been estimated that 70% of the population will have bladder problems at some stage in their lives. There can be many causes of continence problems and help with diagnosis can be given by a GP. In most areas there will be a continence service with specialist advisers.

There are many discreet ways of managing the condition and a continence adviser or a community nurse can give advice. The availability of equipment on the NHS will vary from area to area: some may be free, some available on prescription and some may have to be bought privately. A laundry service or a waste collection service for disposable products may be available.

Advice and support is also available from the following organisations:

Bladder & Bowel Foundation

SATRA Innovation Park, Rockingham Road, Kettering NN16 9JH.
☎ 0870 770 3246.
@ info@bladderandbowelfoundation.org
Ⓦ www.bladderandbowelfoundation.org

Cystitis & Overactive Bladder Foundation

946 Bristol Road South, Northfield, Birmingham B31 2LQ.
☎ 0121 476 1222.
@ info@cobfoundation.org
Ⓦ www.cobfoundation.org

ERIC (Education & Resources for Improving Childhood Continence)

34 Old School House, Britannia Road, Kingswood, Bristol BS15 8DB.
☎ 0117 960 3060.
@ info@eric.org.uk
Ⓦ www.eric.org.uk

PromoCon Information Service

Redbank House, St Chad's Street, Cheetham, Manchester M8 8QA.
☎ 0161 214 5959 or 0161 834 2001 (Confidential Helpline Monday-Friday 10am-3pm).
@ Promocon@disabledliving.co.uk
Ⓦ www.promocon.co.uk

> www.lofric.co.uk is a website for people with urinary problems and bladder disorders. The site, developed by Astra Tech, provides information and advice; particularly, on intermittent self catheterisation.

Continuing Health Care

Many disabled people are now in receipt of a direct payment from their local Social Services Department. This allows them to manage their own care needs, employ personal assistants and become more independent. Some disabled people continue to rely on their social services to provide care directly. Sometimes, particularly with long term conditions where an individual's health may deteriorate over the passage of time, your health related needs may become so paramount that the local authority asks the NHS to support or even inherit your care package. This is known as "continuing care" and will be provided by your local Primary Care Trust (PCT).

The PCT will employ a lead manager, whose responsibility will be to provide and manage continuing care packages. To migrate from part or all of a local authority to NHS paid for care, an assessment will take place. The assessment will determine what proportion of your care needs should be met by the NHS. It is important to remember that care provided by the NHS is free at the point of delivery. Unlike local authority provided care, NHS supported care is not means tested. Thus there is a financial advantage in moving to continuing care where it is appropriate. During the production of this book, the Health Bill was making its way through Parliament. Once that Bill becomes an Act of Parliament, the NHS will be mandated to allow direct payment recipients to migrate their current package unfettered to continuing care where the care is assessed as wholly health related.

Dental Services

If you are unable to visit a dentist, some general dental practitioners will treat you at home if your condition requires this and you are within 5 miles of their practice. Community dental services should provide treatment for those who cannot use general dental services. Information can be obtained from your Primary Care Trust.

Going into and leaving hospital

Key facts

❯ Going into hospital as an inpatient affects your benefits. Some benefits (Attendance Allowance, Disability Living Allowance) can be stopped after a few weeks, while other means-tested benefits may be reduced. Let the offices dealing with you benefits know if you are going into hospital and how long you are likely to stay.

❯ If you have been kept in a psychiatric hospital under the Mental Health Act you are entitled to free after care and support when you leave.

❯ If you have care and support needs you shouldn't be discharged from hospital until proper arrangements and a care plan are in place to ensure you can return home safely without being put at risk of harm. Discharge planning should start early and involve you and any family members/carers you want involved. NHS bodies and local authorities have to work together to ensure this happens. Don't agree to be discharged unless you're happy with the care plan and don't agree to a residential home placement if you're not happy with that (people can find it hard to extricate themselves again). In some areas (Birmingham, for example) there are voluntary services that can provide additional practical support to people coming home from hospital – ask what's available.

❯ If you need a short period of intensive support and rehabilitation to regain your independence on leaving hospital you may get 'intermediate care' (different nations have different terminology - in Wales this is called 6-week support for vulnerable people) - it's free and can last up to 6 weeks; thereafter you should have an assessment to see what ongoing support you need.

Hearing Aid Services

The NHS hearing aid service is free including testing, fitting and servicing. Your GP can refer you to a hospital ear, nose and throat department (ENT) or an audiology department. After an assessment, an appropriate hearing aid is chosen and advice given on how to use it most effectively.

The 2009 RNID Hearing Matters campaign aimed to check the hearing of one million people to persuade the government that 'hearing matters'. A simple 5-minute hearing check is available on 0844 800 3838 or online.

Hearing aids can be bought privately from a registered hearing aid dispenser and this may be quicker and more convenient, although more expensive, than using the NHS.

Hearing Aid Council
70 St Mary Axe, London EC3A 8BE.
☎ 020 3102 4030. @ hac@thehearingaidcouncil.org.uk
Ⓦ www.thehearingaidcouncil.org.uk

The HAC, a statutory body, can provide a list of registered hearing aid dispensers so that consumers can check if they are using a dispenser that meets certain standards of conduct. If necessary it can provide a complaints procedure.

Hearing therapists provide advice support and help to anyone with difficulty communicating because of a hearing problem. They can show people how to use their remaining hearing most effectively. Referral is often after attending an ENT or Hearing Aid Clinic.

British Academy of Audiology

Association House, South Park Road, Macclesfield SK11 6SH.

☎ 01625 504066. @ admin@baaudiology.org

Ⓦ www.baaudiology.org

BAA represents different groups of people working within audiology with the intention of becoming a professional body.

Occupational Therapy

Occupational therapists (OTs), who may work in social services or the NHS, use practical means to promote independence. They can assess ability to undertake everyday activities such as bathing, dressing and getting around and advise on suitable home adaptations and equipment. OTs can also be helpful in assisting people to participate in social and other activities. People may be referred to an OT by a hospital consultant or GP or they may refer themselves to the social services department.

British Association/College of Occupational Therapists

College of Occupational Therapists, 106-114 Borough High Street, London SE1 1LB.

☎ 020 7357 6480. Ⓦ www.baot.co.uk

The professional and representative body for occupational therapists can provide information on OTs in private practice.

Optical Services

NHS eye tests not only assess the current state of your vision but will normally include an examination for the early signs of other sight problems and some other conditions such as diabetes. Eye tests are free if you are:

❯ Aged 60 or over, under 16 or under 19 and in full-time education;

❯ Are claiming certain income related benefits;

❯ Have diabetes or glaucoma, or are over 40 with a close relative who has glaucoma;

❯ Have a low income certificate;

❯ Are registered blind or partially sighted.

If you cannot visit an optician unaccompanied, you can arrange for a home visit. This may be carried out or arranged through a local optician or by self-referral to a specialist organisation.

The Outside Clinic provides a national, domiciliary optician service. Its optometrists who make home visits by appointment are equipped to detect glaucoma, cataracts and other potential problems as well as testing eyesight and advising on the choice of spectacles. On a second appointment the glasses are delivered and fitted. An aftercare service and repeat appointments are offered. The service is offered on NHS terms. For further information contact The Outside Clinic, Old Town Court, 10-14 High Street, Swindon SN1 3EP. ☎ 0800 854 477. @ info@outsideclinic.com ⓦ www.outsideclinic.com

The General Optical Council
41 Harley Street, London W1G 8DJ.

☎ 020 7580 3898. @ goc@optical.org ⓦ www.optical.org

The GOC is the statutory body that regulates the optical professions in the UK. It maintains a register of people who have adequate training, practical experience and qualification to practice as dispensing opticians and optometrists and manages matters relating to optical training and examinations. Complaints from members of the public about members of the optical profession are considered by the GOC's disciplinary system, which can lead to an optician being removed from the register.

The Federation of Ophthalmic and Dispensing Opticians
99 Gloucester Terrace, London W2 6LD.

☎ 020 7298 5151. @ info@fodo.com ⓦ www.fodo.com

FODO represents opticians in their business interests whether as individuals, family firms or chains. It has issued guidance to its members on improving facilities and services for disabled people at their premises and hosts the Domiciliary Eye Care Committee.

Pharmacy

In addition to dispensing prescribed drugs and selling medicines that do not require a prescription, pharmacists or chemists can be a useful source of information on a range of health matters. They may be more convenient to visit than a GP.

Royal Pharmaceutical Society of GB

1 Lambeth High Street, London SE1 7JN.

☎ 020 7735 9141. @ enquiries@rpsgb.org ⓦ www.rpsgb.org.uk

The professional and regulatory body for pharmacists in England, Scotland and Wales.

Physiotherapy

Physiotherapy aims to improve movement, strength and function by using a range of treatments including exercise, manipulation, heat, light and sound. Physiotherapists work widely in hospitals and also in community settings, often as part of a multidisciplinary rehabilitation team, to enable sick or disabled people to function as well as possible. Some areas have domiciliary physiotherapists who do home visits and there are also physiotherapists who work privately, some of whom undertake specialist services, for example treating sports injuries.

The Chartered Society of Physiotherapy

14 Bedford Row, London WC1R 4ED.

☎ 020 7306 6666. ⓦ www.csp.org.uk

CSP is the professional organisation for physiotherapists representing those with a recognised qualification. Physiotherapists in private practice can be found on the Physio2u pages of its website.

Prescriptions

There are a number of ways of reducing or avoiding your spend on prescriptions. If you do not qualify for free prescriptions and have an average of two or more prescriptions/month, it will almost certainly be cheaper to buy a quarterly or annual "season ticket". This enables you to pay a set fee for three or twelve months. During the paid for period, all prescriptions will be free. Ask your pharmacist for more details.

Additionally, people with some specific long term and other conditions now qualify for free prescriptions – for example, people with cancer, people with a physical condition that makes it impossible to attend the pharmacy and so on. Your GP or your pharmacist can tell you more.

Speech and Language Therapy

Speech and language therapists treat children and adults with communications difficulties from a wide range of causes. The therapist, after assessment, will advise on a programme to maximise communications skill, if necessary using methods such as signing or technological aids. Help with certain swallowing and feeding problems may also be available.

Royal College of Speech & Language Therapists
2 White Hart Yard, London SE1 1NX.
☎ 020 7378 1200. Ⓦ www.rcslt.org

The professional body for speech and language therapists.

HOLIDAYS

First of all, decide on the type of holiday you want. This will include whether you want to go on your own, with family and friends or if you prefer an organised group of some kind. It will also include the choice of staying where meals are provided or in self-catering accommodation; which general area you want to visit and what you want to do when you get there.

It may be possible to find out quite a lot of information about the destination area. General local tourist guides and other publications will often give an indication of suitability and sometimes more specific information for disabled visitors. Access Guides exist for some towns. The Tourist Information Centre is likely to be a good source of information as may be a disability organisation local to the area.

Tourism for All

c/o Vitalise, Shap Road Industrial Estate, Kendal LA9 6NZ.
☎ 0845 124 9971. Textphone: 0845 124 9976.
Ⓦ www.tourismforall.org.uk

Tourism for All, previously known as Holiday Care, is UK's central source of holiday and travel information for disabled and older people and carers. Information can be given on accessible accommodation, visitor attractions and transport, both in the UK and at some overseas destinations and identifies sources of funding for disabled people on low incomes. Tourism for All also works with all sectors of the tourism industry to improve accessibility and carries out inspections under the National Accessible Scheme.

Booking

Whether a holiday is booked independently, direct with the accommodation or through a tour operator, think through whether you want to specify your requirements and if so what exactly you want to ask for. You are the expert on this but some accommodation providers and tour operators may be inclined to make assumptions about you. It may be annoying to be asked apparently irrelevant questions, but this can better than not being asked anything.

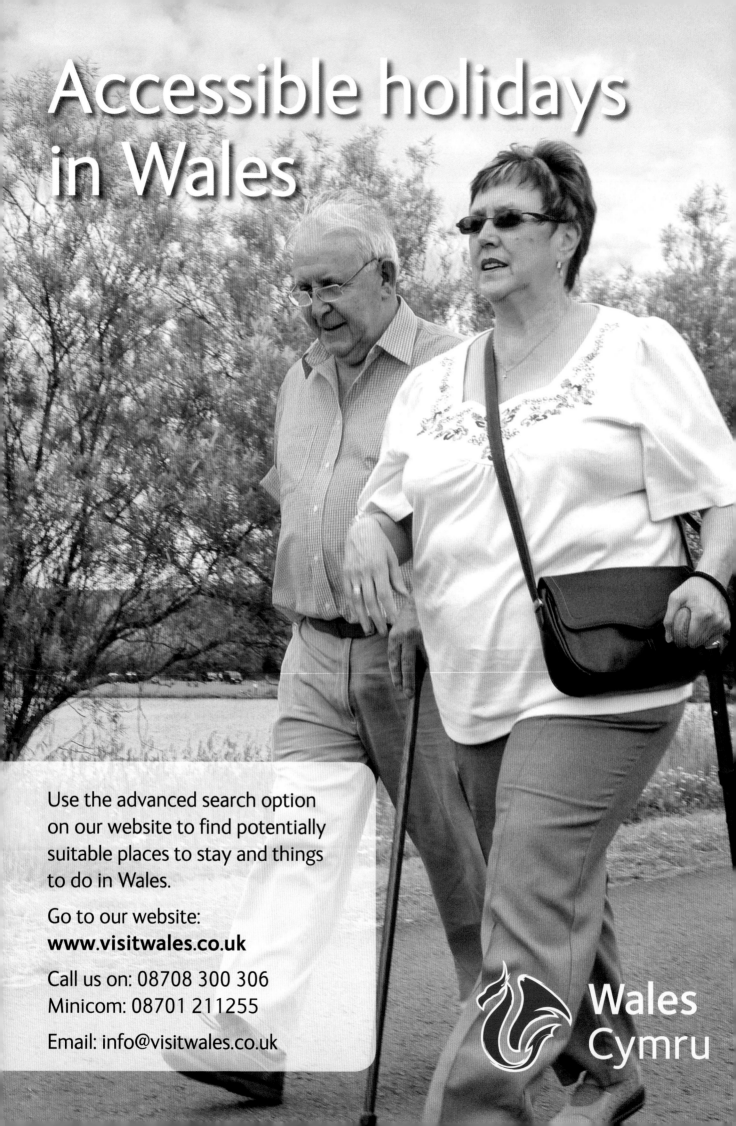

It can be valuable to prepare a list of the facilities that you want at the destination and useful to divide these between those which are absolutely essential and those which are desirable. Facilities may include the physical accessibility of the premises and surroundings, the availability of equipment and appropriate transport and the provision of assistance or other services.

You may have to make arrangements for transport to and from your destination. Even if a major part of the journey is included in the package, the first and last bits of the trip will normally be your responsibility. For further information see the chapter on Public Transport.

Travelling Abroad

There are a number of points to consider before travelling overseas. The first is that attitudes, services and legislation relating to disability will be different. They may be better or worse in all or some respects but they will be different. Many voluntary organisations dealing with specific conditions can advise their members on overseas travel.

Medical treatment – If you become ill or have an accident abroad, you will probably have to pay for all or part of your treatment. This is a major reason for ensuring that you have adequate insurance for the full period of the holiday. Health Advice for Travellers, a leaflet issued by the Department of Health and available from Post Offices and other information points, gives much information on health and medical treatment in other countries. It also contains a form for the European Health Insurance Card (EHIC) that is required to make use of the reciprocal health agreements that the UK has with a number of countries, particularly in the European Union. The EHIC card is valid for 5 years, so holders should check the expiry date of their card in advance of travelling.

Regular Medication – If you use, or are likely to require any regularly prescribed medicines, dressings, etc, make sure you take an adequate supply with you, including enough for any unforeseen delays. These should be packed in hand luggage. This is so that they are available during the journey and so that they can readily be explained to Customs or Immigration officials. It may be useful to have a note from your GP explaining your need for them. Any liquids or gels should be in their original packaging from the chemist, especially if you are flying.

Passports – The Identity & Passport Service offers assistance with completing passport applications whether on paper or online. Braille and audio information are available. Regional and other offices used for face-to-face interviews with new passport applicants are accessible and have staff who can use sign language. Contact The Passport Adviceline ☎ 0300 222 0000. Textphone: 0300 222 0222. ⓦ www.ips.gov.uk

Insurance

It is essential to take out adequate insurance for a holiday. Although travel insurance is generally associated with overseas travel, it is also available and should be considered for holidays in the UK as well.

In many countries the cost of medical treatment in the event of illness or accident has to be met in full and can be frighteningly high. Even in countries with which Britain has reciprocal health care agreements, part of the cost of treatment often has to be paid. Insurance may also be required to cover the cost of property that is damaged or lost while on holiday, to recoup money if the holiday has to be cancelled or cut short or to provide some compensation for delays.

While any blanket refusal to provide insurance cover, or charge higher rates, for disabled people is unlawful there can still be difficulties or higher costs for some people. It is worth checking whether a standard policy offered by a travel company meets your own needs. Some voluntary organisations can assist their members, or people with the condition with which they are concerned, to obtain appropriate cover.

Companies with insurance packages designed for disabled people include:

AllClear Travel Insurance
6th Floor, Regents House,
Hubert Road, Brentwood CM14 4JE.
☎ 0871 208 8579.
@ info@allcleartravel.co.uk
ⓦ www.allcleartravel.co.uk

En Route Insurance
Grove Mills, Cranbrook Road,
Hawkhurst, Kent TN18 4AS.
☎ 0800 783 7245.
@ info@enrouteinsurance.co.uk
ⓦ www.enrouteinsurance.co.uk

Chartwell Insurance
Chartwell House, 229-294
Hale Lane, Edgware HA8 8NP.
☎ 0845 260 7051/2.
@ info@chartwellinsurance.co.uk
ⓦ www.chartwellinsurance.co.uk

Fogg Travel Insurance Services Ltd
Crow Hill Drive, Mansfield NG19 7AE.
☎ 01623 631331.
@ sales@fogginsure.co.uk
ⓦ www.fogginsure.co.uk

Free Spirit
P J Hayman & Company Ltd,
Stansted House, Rowlands Castle,
Hampshire PO9 6DX.
☎ 0845 230 5000.
@ freesprit@pjhayman.com
Ⓦ www.free-spirit.com

Travelbility
Peregrine House, Bakers Lane, Epping
CM16 5DQ.
☎ 0845 338 1638.
@ enquiries@travelbility.co.uk
Ⓦ www.travelbility.co.uk

Voluntary Organisations

Many of the voluntary organisations dealing with specific disabilities or which operate on a local basis give advice on holidays and/or arrange holidays for their members. Some, including the Multiple Sclerosis Society and Action for Blind People, have their own holiday accommodation. In addition the following organisations make holiday provision more widely for disabled people.

3H Fund
B2 Speldhurst Business Park, Langton Road, Speldhurst,
Tunbridge Wells TN3 0AQ.
☎ 01892 860207.
@ info@3hfund.org.uk
Ⓦ www.3hfund.org.uk

The 3H Fund provides subsidised group holidays for physically disabled people, from 11 years upwards, who would otherwise be unable to take a break. Holidays are inclusive of accommodation and transport and groups include experienced volunteers and nursing staff provide help. The programme includes weeks in Britain and abroad.

Holidays for Disabled People
PO Box 164, Totton, Southampton
SO40 9WZ.
@ disholspw@aol.com
Ⓦ www.holidaqysfordisabled.com

A group holiday on the Norfolk Coast is offered for disabled people each year. Volunteer helpers are available and there is a nursing/medical presence in the group.

Holidays with Help
4 Pebblecombe, Adelaide Road,
Surbiton, Surrey KT6 4LL.
☎ 020 8390 9752.
Ⓦ www.holidayswithhelp.org.uk

Holidays with Help runs group holidays for disabled people at holiday centres in England. Activities and outings are arranged. Experienced helpers and medical and nursing personnel are available. Applications accepted from groups, families and individuals. Apply to Rosemary McIntyre at the above address.

Livability Holidays

50 Scrutton Street,
London EC2A 4XQ.
☎ 020 7452 2000.
@ holidays@livability.org.uk
Ⓦ www.livability.org.uk

Livability, previously John Grooms and Shaftesbury, offers a range of holiday accommodation including hotels at Minehead and Llandudno and self-catering units around England and Wales including units at holiday parks and self-contained houses and flats equipped for disabled holidaymakers.

Papillon Holidays

1 Exeter Drive, Ashton-under-Lyne
OL6 8BZ.
☎ 0774 959 8423.
Ⓦ www.papillonholidays.co.uk

Papillon Holidays offers a range of holidays throughout the year with support in Britain particularly for adults with learning and physical disabilities.

Scout Holiday Homes Trust

Gilwell Park, Bury Road, Chingford,
London E4 7QW.
☎ 020 8433 7290.
@ lynda.peters@scout.org.uk
Ⓦ www.scoutbase.org.uk/hq/holhomes

SHHT offers low cost self-catering holidays in 6-berth chalets and caravans with some adaptations at a number of holiday parks around the English and Welsh coasts. Any family with a disabled member welcomed - not only those in Scouting. The season is generally from Easter-October and bookings are taken from the previous October.

Vitalise

Shap Road Industrial Estate,
Shap Road, Kendal LA9 6NZ.
☎ 0845 330 0149.
Ⓦ www.vitalise.org.uk

Vitalise provides breaks for disabled people at 5 accessible centres in Cornwall, Essex, Hampshire, Nottinghamshire and Southport. Each provides 24-hour care on-call and personal support. Theme weeks for specific interests and age groups are arranged, including several special Alzheimer's and MS Society weeks each year. It also runs Holidays for Visually Impaired People accompanied by volunteer sighted companions and can arrange overseas holidays for disabled people at selected accessible hotels.

Specialist Commercial Organisations

The following organisations specialise in offering holidays and related services to disabled people:

Accessatlast Ltd

18 Hazel Grove, Tarleton,
Preston PR4 6DQ.
☎ 01772 814555.
Ⓦ www.accessatlast.com

Company founded by a wheelchair user whose website gives information on hotel and self-catering accommodation in many countries.

Access Travel

6 The Hillock, Astley, Lancashire
M29 7GW.
☎ 01942 888844.
@ info@access-travel.co.uk
Ⓦ www.access-travel.co.uk

Offers a programme of holiday packages designed for disabled people in the Mediterranean, the Canaries and Florida. Sailing among the Greek Islands and holiday homes in France are also offered. A variety of self-catering and hotel accommodations are available.

Accessible Travel & Leisure

Avionics House, Naas Lane, Quedgeley, Gloucester GL2 4SN.

☎ 01452 729739.

@ info@accessibletravel.co.uk

Ⓦ www.accessibletravel.co.uk

A specialist travel service that offers a wide range of holidays and related services for disabled people including Mediterranean holidays, cruises and tours in South Africa and Egypt. Accessible villas, apartments and hotels are offered together with accessible transfers or car hire, local representatives and insurance.

ATS Travel Ltd

1 Tank Lane, Purfleet, Essex RM16 1TA.

☎ 01708 863198.

@ aatstravel@aol.com

Ⓦ www.assistedholidays.com

Arranges holidays for disabled people and their families in Britain and abroad. Accessible accommodation is used and transport, trips and holiday insurance can be arranged. A variety of hotel, self-catering and touring are offered.

Can Be Done Ltd

11 Woodcock Hill, Harrow HA3 0XP.

☎ 020 8907 2400.

@ holidays@canbedone.co.uk

Ⓦ www.canbedone.co.uk

Can Be Done, a tour operator founded by a wheelchair user, offers holidays for people with access or mobility problems. Its programme includes a wide range of destinations in Britain, Ireland, continental Europe and other destinations throughout the world but tailor-made holidays and tours can be arranged anywhere.

Chalfont Line

4 Providence Road, West Drayton UB7 8HJ.

☎ 01895 459540.

Ⓦ www.chalfont-line.co.uk

Chalfont Line, a long-established adapted coach hire company, has a programme of leisurely paced holidays for wheelchair users and others with impaired mobility in Britain and overseas. A door-to-door service and personal assistance can be provided at extra cost.

Diana's Supported Holidays

18 Parish Close, Broadstairs CT10 2UJ

☎ 0844 800 9373.

@ enquiries@dsh.org.uk

Ⓦ www.dsh.org.uk

Holidays with support are offered for people with learning disabilities at seaside resorts and countryside areas in Britain and a number destinations abroad. Groups are of at least six with a qualified leader and support staff. Up to one-to-one support can be arranged if required although a lower ratio is normally provided. In addition to the programmed holidays, other destinations can be arranged for groups.

Enable Holidays Ltd

The Green, Kings Norton, Birmingham B38 8SD.

☎ 0871 222 4939.

@ info@enableholidays.com

Ⓦ www.enableholidays.com

This company offers package holidays at selected resorts in the Mediterranean, The Canaries and Florida at hotels chosen as being accessible. Powered wheelchairs and other equipment can be pre-booked and adapted vehicles arranged for transfers and outings in many locations.

Katalan Travels

☎ 01494 580816.

@ katalan.travels@ntlworld.com

Ⓦ www.holidayswithaccess.com

A travel company offering a specialist holiday consultancy and booking service for disabled people, whether travelling individually, in families or larger groups. All aspects of any type of holiday in Britain or worldwide can be covered including transport, transfers, accommodation, insurance, equipment hire and care services.

Traveleyes

PO Box 511, Leeds LS5 3JT.

☎ 0870 922 0221. Ⓦ www.traveleyes. co.uk

Travel company organising small group holidays for visually impaired and sighted people, with the latter acting as guides in exchange for a discounted price. Holidays have included walking trips in southern Spain and the Atlas mountains, visits to Malta and Morocco and activity breaks in southern Africa. Groups are kept to around 15.

Wings on Wheels

8 Cornfields, Church Lane, Tydd St Giles, Wisbech PE13 5LX.

☎ 01945 871111.

@ info@wingsonwheels.co.uk

Ⓦ www.wingsonwheels.co.uk

Offer a programme of escorted holidays for disabled and non-disabled people throughout the year to destinations in Europe and further afield.

www.matchinghouses.com
A website for disabled people who wish to house-swap for their holidays based on the principle that if an exchange can be arranged between people with similar access needs they should both be able to travel with greater confidence within this country or further afield.

HOUSING

If you begin to find it difficult to get around your home, you may well be entitled to help from your local authority to adapt it to your needs or to find a more accessible place to live.

This section tells you about:

❯ your rights to adaptations

❯ things to think about if you need to move home

❯ when you can get help with paying your mortgage

❯ how the Disability Discrimination Act protects you against discrimination by landlords and people selling property

❯ help available to insulate your home and cut energy costs.

❯ sheltered housing options

House Adaptations

Most areas have a 'Home improvement service' to help disabled and older people with quick repairs and small adaptations like grab rails. They can also help get grants for bigger adaptations (see below). Many also offer 'handy person services' to do small jobs in the home, put in safety features and help make sure homes are suitable for people to return to after a spell in hospital. In 2009-10 the Government plans to expand and improve these services because they are such great value for money.

To find out where your nearest home improvement service is contact:

Foundations
Bleaklow House, Howard Town Mill, Glossop SK13 8NT.
☎ 01457 891909. Ⓦ www.foundations.uk.com

For bigger adaptations – a downstairs shower-room, wider doorways or an adapted kitchen – you could apply to your local housing authority for a Disabled Facilities Grant (DFG).

Disabled homeowners and tenants have a legal right to a Disabled Facilities Grant for adaptations needed to:

❯ Make it easier to get into and out of the home, for example by widening doors or building a ramp;

❯ Improve access to the garden;

❯ Ensure your safety and that of other people living with you, for example by improved lighting or providing a specially adapted room where someone can be left unattended;

❯ Improve access to the living room and bedroom;

❯ Provide or improve access to the kitchen, toilet, washbasin and bath or shower, for example by providing a stairlift or installing a downstairs bathroom;

❯ Improve or provide a suitable heating system and adapt heating and lighting controls to make them easier to use;

❯ Improve access and movement around the home so you can care for another resident, such as a child or spouse.

The DFG is administered by local housing authorities. To approve a grant they must be satisfied that the works are necessary and appropriate for the needs of the disabled person as well as being reasonable and practicable in relation to the property. You'll usually be assessed by an occupational therapist. They will then make a recommendation to the housing grants officers.

Once you have filled in the formal application form you are entitled to a decision within 6 months.

The maximum grant payable is £30,000 in England, Wales and Northern Ireland. There is no financial means test for disabled children under 19. However, disabled adults will face a means-test. How big a contribution you will be asked to make towards the works will depend on you and your partner's income and capital.

If you are having building work done

❯ Check if you need planning permission beforehand – most common building works and extensions won't but you must check.

- You or your builder also need to ensure work complies with building regulations.

- If it's a big project, use a qualified architect or surveyor to prepare the plans and supervise the work.

- Check the reputation of any builders and contractors and ensure that they are members of a trade association, such as the Federation of Master Builders or the National Federation of Builders that provides a guarantee or arbitration service.

- See if your local authority has a list of architects, surveyors, builders and others who have experience of carrying out adaptations in the area.

VAT on building work

Some building work to make housing meet the needs of a disabled occupant can be zero rated for VAT. This includes:

- Building ramps or widening doorways or passages in your home (but not building new ones)

- Extending or adapting a bathroom or loo

- Installing a lift in your home so you can move between floors

- Putting in an alarm system so you can call for help

The contractor or supplier should know about this and information is available in VAT Notice 701/7 from HM Revenue and Customs.

You can get more advice about all of this from your local authority, a housing advice centre, Home Improvement Agency or Citizens Advice Bureau or online at www.direct.gov.uk.

A booklet, **Disabled Facilities Grant**, can be downloaded from the Department of Communities & Local Government website www.communities.gov.uk. For copies in alternative formats email alternativeformats@communities.gsi.gov.uk quoting the title or the following product code: 9781409810469, as well as your address and telephone number.

Other Financial Assistance

Housing authorities also have the power to provide discretionary assistance that might be used to top-up a Disabled Facilities Grant or to help people move if this would be a better option. They might provide low cost loans or equity release schemes for private householders.

Social Services also have legal duties to help disabled people with adaptations. This is useful if you need an adaptation which costs more than the maximum DFG grant, or you can't afford the contribution you'd need to make under DFG. Social services also usually provide equipment and adaptations costing up to £1,000 for which you cannot be charged. They can also lend you things like stairlifts.

Moving home

There are many reasons for wanting to move home; the current one may not be suitable for adaptation or for current family needs or you may want to move to a different area or you may be seeking a home for the first time.

If you can't afford to buy and you have a low income contact your local authority about going on the housing register.   This is a list of people who want to rent council or housing association properties. Since there are more people in need than there are homes available, councils have to prioritise. Anyone who needs to move for medical or access reasons should get additional priority – but check out your council's policies on this in detail.

In England many local authorities have adopted 'Choice-based lettings' which means people on the housing register are not offered a particular property, they are invited to 'bid' for any available property they think meets their needs. Properties with access features should be flagged up. Whose bid is successful depends on who has the biggest priority need.

Some areas have a dedicated Disabled Person's Housing Service that can offer individual advice and/or an **Accessible Housing Register** with up to date details of accessible or adapted homes available for renting.

Councils have powers to pay a 'relocation grant' to help someone move to a home which is already more accessible or could be made so more easily.

Some **housing associations** have their own waiting lists so it's also worth contacting them directly. Housing associations are non-profit organisations providing rented homes or assistance for people on low-incomes to buy their own homes. Some operate on a local or regional basis across the range of housing requirements and others specialise in providing housing for people with particular housing needs, such as forms of supported housing.

Most Housing Association vacancies are filled by people nominated by the local authority of the area. However, depending on their individual policies, they may also accept applications from individuals or from other organisations. Some Associations operate partnership schemes with voluntary bodies in which they provide the housing with the partner providing an agreed level of care or support for the tenants.

Housing associations often run **shared ownership** schemes. Shared-ownership is when you part buy and part rent a home. You might buy a 25%, 50% or 75% share in your home and pay a small rent on the share that you don't buy. For more information go to www.shared-ownership.org.uk. The Government also has a scheme for first time buyers, key workers and social tenants called Home Buy. More details are available at www.homebuy.org.uk.

If you are considering buying a newly built house, it is well worth

❯ checking what accessibility standards it is built to and/or

❯ contacting the developer to see if any design features that are required can be built in.

All new homes are supposed to be built to standards that enable disabled people, particularly wheelchair users and people with mobility impairments, to visit a house and have access to a ground floor living space and toilet. Increasing numbers (mainly social housing) are being built to the Lifetime Homes standards.

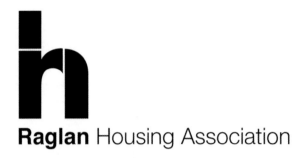
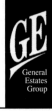

Lifetime Homes is a popular design concept that makes new housing accessible for disabled people and easy to adapt in the future to meet individual requirements that may emerge. The concept has been adopted by a number of social housing providers but so far by few private housebuilders. The Government has announced that all social housing is to be built to the Lifetime Homes standards by 2011. Private housebuilders are expected to adopt the standard by 2013 or will face new regulation forcing them to do it.

The features of Lifetime Homes include:

⊙ Level entry to the main entrance, or a suitable alternative;

⊙ An entrance door wide enough to allow for wheelchair access;

⊙ A toilet on the entrance level that is capable of having a shower installed;

⊙ Adequate circulation and door widths in the entrance floor;

⊙ Switches, sockets and other controls at appropriate heights;

⊙ Level or gently sloping path from a nearby parking space to the dwelling entrance;

⊙ Where a lift of appropriate size is provided in blocks of flats;

⊙ Walls and ceilings to which handrails and hoists can be fitted in bathrooms and adjoining bedrooms;

⊙ An area that could be used as a bedroom on the entrance floor;

⊙ Staircases of a design that will facilitate the fitting of a stairlift or space for a through-floor lift.

If you need a wheelchair accessible home – a home with the necessary circulation space and level access to provide full wheelchair access to all parts of the home – it's worth checking with local housing associations. Also try the Accessible Property Register (details below). RADAR is pressing for more wheelchair accessible housing, there's a real shortage at the moment.

Help with mortgage payments

If you start to get behind with your mortgage payments it's important to get advice from your bank or mortgage lender as soon as possible. You may be able to make arrangements to renegotiate the terms of your repayments. Your lender should treat you fairly and think about what they can do to help you keep your home. You can also get advice from Citizens Advice.

In England there is a new **Mortgage Rescue Scheme** (with similar schemes planned in Wales, Scotland and Northern Ireland) for people who are at risk of becoming homeless because they're unexpectedly unable to meet their mortgage repayments. This scheme is for people with 'priority needs' including disabled people whose household income is less than £60,000 a year. Check out if you are eligible by contacting your local housing authority.

There is also a **Homeowner Mortgage Support Scheme** to help homeowners who suffer a temporary fall in income but who are expected to recover at a later date.

People claiming certain means-tested benefits (pension credit, income-based Jobseekers Allowance, Income Support) can **get help with mortgage interest payments.** From January 2009 people making new claims to benefits are entitled to get help with their eligible mortgage interest after 13 weeks of being unemployed (rather than 39 weeks). This help is available on an increased capital amount of up to £200,000 (rather than the previous £100,000 limit). These changes will be reviewed once housing market conditions improve.

Housing and the DDA

The Disability Discrimination Act makes it unlawful for anyone letting, selling or managing rented property to discriminate against disabled people. So landlords cannot refuse to let a flat to you, evict or harass you, offer you a lease on worse terms or stop you using facilities everyone else has access to for a reason relating to your disability. Landlords also have to make reasonable adjustments, for example: providing tenancy agreements in an accessible format or waiving a 'no-animals' term in a lease so you can keep an assistance dog. Although they aren't required to change physical features, they do need to consider changing things like signs, doorbells and taps so they are easier to use.

Landlords are not allowed to refuse you permission, unreasonably, to make bigger changes to the property which you need because of a disability. You will have to pay for the alterations yourself or get a grant. This right does not yet apply to 'common parts' – that is, to hallways or stairs. In Scotland, the right does apply to the 'common parts' but the other tenants need to agree to the change too, as does the landlord.

Warm Front Grants

The Government funded Warm Front scheme (Ⓦ www.warmfront.co.uk, ☎ 0800 316 2805) provides a grant for heating and insulation improvements to householders across England. Similar schemes are available in Scotland, Wales and Northern Ireland. Eligible households include people who own their home or rent from a private landlord and receive certain benefits. The scheme is specifically designed to assist those people most vulnerable to cold related problems and includes: people with disabilities and long term illnesses, older people, families with young children and expectant mothers who are in receipt of income or disability related benefits. A package of heating and insulation measures will be prepared and managed to meet individual needs and may include loft insulation, cavity wall insulation, draught proofing and central heating. People over 60 who do not receive any of the benefits for the full scheme can apply for a discount on the cost of installing central heating, although funds for this are limited.

For further information contact Eaga Partnership, Eaga House, Archbold Terrace, Newcastle upon Tyne NE2 1DB. ☎ 0800 316 2805. @ enquiry@eaga.com Ⓦ www.eaga.com

For further free, impartial advice on energy saving in your home and cutting your fuel bills you can contact the Energy Saving Trust. ☎ 0800 512 012. www.energysavingtrust.org.uk

Sheltered housing

If you want housing with extra support and security but don't want to forego your independence, there are a growing range of options.

Sheltered housing, often but not exclusively provided for older people, comes in the form of a group of appropriately designed self-contained flats or houses with 24-hour emergency assistance plus the security of having a warden on hand. There are usually communal facilities – like a lounge and gardens. Some schemes are developed with additional care services being provided – this is often called "Extra Care Housing". Most sheltered housing is for rent and available through your local authority or housing association. Increasingly, private developers and a number of housing associations are offering a variety of purchase options for you to buy your own property.

AIMS

Age Concern England, Astral House, 1268 London Road, London SW16 4ER.
@ 0845 600 2001(Helpline) or 020 8765 7465. @ aims@ace.org.uk
Ⓦ www.ageconcern.org.uk

AIMS (Advice, Information and Mediation Service) is a specialist service offering impartial information, advice and mediation for anyone who lives in or is involved in providing private retirement or rented sheltered housing.

Elderly Accommodation Counsel

3rd Floor, 89 Albert Embankment, London SE1 7TP.
@ 020 7820 1343.
@ enquiries@eac.org.uk
Ⓦ www.housingcare.org

EAC maintains a register of sheltered housing schemes which is available on the above website and can advise elderly people on all matters related to accommodation and related care.

ERoSH

PO Box 2616,Chippenham, Wiltshire SN15 1WZ.
@ 01249 654 249.
@ info@shelteredhousing.org
Ⓦ www.shelteredhousing.org

EroSH is the national consortium for sheltered and retirement housing and publishes "An Essential Guide to Sheltered Housing". It works on behalf of older people and sheltered housing providers to improve housing and support for existing and future sheltered housing residents.

Other Useful Contacts

Accessible Property Register

c/o Conrad Hodgkinson, 11 Stumperlowe Croft, Sheffield S10 3QW.
@ 0774 9119 385.
@ conradh@accessible-property.org.uk
Ⓦ www.accessible-property.org.uk

The Accessible Property website gives information on accessible and adapted housing for sale or rent, including both private and social housing. Advertisements from private individuals are free and people who are looking for housing can place a 'Property Wanted' notice.

Counsel and Care

Twyman House, 16 Bonny Street, London NW1 6PG.
@ 020 7241 8555.
@ advice@counselandcare.org.uk
Ⓦ www.counselandcare.org.uk

Counsel and Care provides information and advice for elderly people and their families and carers on residential and community care. It has published The Complete Care Home Guide and The Brief Care Home Guide, both of which together with a number of factsheets are available free of charge from the above address or can be downloaded from the website.

Habinteg Housing Association

Holyer House, 20-21 Red Lion Court, London EC4A 3EB.
@ 020 7822 8700.
@ info@habinteg.org.uk
ⓦ www.habinteg.org.uk

One of leading specialist providers of accessible housing, Habinteg provides over 2000 homes across England of which over a quarter are designed for wheelchair users and the rest to accessibility standards. It also operates in Northern Ireland, Scotland, Wales and the Irish Republic through sister organisations. Habinteg also played a major part in developing the "Lifetime Homes" concept.

Housing Ombudsman Service

81 Aldwych, London WC2B 4HN.
@ 0845 712 5973.
Textphone: 020 7404 7092.
@ info@housing-ombudsman.org.uk
ⓦ www.ihos.org.uk

This independent organisation can take up complaints from residents of housing provided by social landlords, including those who have taken over properties from local authorities, and a number of other organisations that have joined HOS. People should have used their landlord's own complaints procedure before registering with HOS. Local authority tenants should contact the Local Government Ombudsman. The Housing Ombudsman only operates in England.

Housing Options

Stanelaw House, Sutton Lane, Sutton, Witney OX29 5RY.
@ 0845 456 1497.
@ enquiries@housingoptions.org.uk
ⓦ www.housingoptions.org.uk

Housing Options provides an advisory service for anyone concerned with housing for people with learning disabilities, their families and carers. The website includes a wide range of information sheets.

Livability

50 Scrutton Street, London EC2A 4XQ.
@ 020 7452 2000.
@ info@livability.org.uk
ⓦ www.livability.org.uk

Livability specialises in homes designed and adapted for wheelchair users and their families in order to enable independence. Livability also provides a wide range of accessible holiday accommodation for disabled people.

Joseph Rowntree Foundation

The Homestead, 40 Water End, York YO30 6WP.
@ 01904 629241.
@ info@jrf.org.uk
ⓦ www.jrf.org.uk

The Joseph Rowntree Foundation is the UK's largest independent social policy research and development charity. It supports a wide programme of research and development projects in housing, social care and social policy. The Foundation also carries out practical innovative projects in housing and care through the Joseph Rowntree Housing Trust including the development of the concept of Lifetime Homes.

Mobility Friendly Homes

99 South Street, Eastbourne BN21 4LU.

@ 0845 612 0280.

@ info@mobilityfriendlyhomes.co.uk

Ⓦ www.mobilityfriendlyhomes.co.uk

This organisation is an internet estate agent service for disabled people seeking to buy or rent a house or flat. Properties from across the UK are listed geographically giving details of access features and adaptations as well as other property details.

National Housing Federation

Lion Court, 25 Procter Street, London WC1V 6NY.

@ 020 7067 1010.

Ⓦ www.housing.org.uk

The NHF represents and can provide information on Housing Associations and other independent social landlords and affordable housing providers in England. It has around 1300 members who are responsible for 2 million homes. The NHF has issued Level Threshold to its members advising on services and approaches that should be provided to disabled people.

For other parts of the UK contact:

Northern Ireland Federation of Housing Associations

38 Hill Street, Belfast BT1 2LB.

@ 028 9023 0446.

Ⓦ www.nifha.org

Scottish Federation of Housing Associations

Pegasus House, 375 West George Street, Glasgow G2 4LW.

@ 0141 332 8113.

Ⓦ www.sfha.co.uk

Community Housing Cymru

Fulmar House, Beignon Close, Ocean Park, Cardiff CF24 5HF.

@ 029 2055 7400.

Ⓦ www.chcymru.org.uk

Ownership Options in Scotland The John Cotton Centre, 10 Sunnyside, Edinburgh EH7 5RA.

@ 0131 661 3400

Ⓦ www.ownershipoptions.org.uk

Ownership Options is a charity established to provide information and advice to disabled people in Scotland to help them overcome the legal, financial and practical barriers to home ownership.

Shelter

88 Old Street, London EC1V 9HU.

@ 0845 458 4590.

@ info@shelter.org.uk

Ⓦ www.shelter.org.uk

Shelter campaigns for decent housing and helps people find and keep a home. It provides advice by telephone, publications, on its website and through a network of housing advice centres around the country. The advice Helpline is open from 8am-8pm every day on 0808 800 4444.

INDEPENDENT LIVING

Disabled people have a human right to support for independent living. Independent living means having the practical support you need to live in the community, have a full life and have a real say over how that support is arranged and provided. Usually this support is referred to as 'community care' or 'social care' and it is your local authority's responsibility to provide this. This section provides a brief guide to your rights, how to go about getting support and what to do if you don't feel you are getting the help you need. It also tells you about direct payments and individual budgets which are ways you can take more control over care and support services. Often people need long-term healthcare as part of their support package, so we also explain about that too.

It can often feel like a bit of battle to get the support you need, so there are details of organisations which can help with more information and support at the end.

Many people buy and arrange their own support, without the local authority's help - brief advice is offered below on how to find out what your options are and things to think about.

Step one: assessment of need for community care

The first thing you need to do is ask social services for an assessment of your needs. In England there are different departments for 'Adult social care' and 'Children's Services'. Disabled people (of any age) have the legal right to such an assessment.

Social services are supposed to take a holistic view of your needs and involve you in the process (often it doesn't feel like that!). If you have housing or health needs they are supposed to get information and assistance from the housing department and the Primary Care Trust/ Local Health Board. You can have a friend or advocate with you for your assessment.

Older people are supposed to receive a 'single assessment' that looks at social care, health and other needs so you don't have to go through lots of different assessments with different agencies, but that doesn't always happen.

An assessment is supposed to look at the ability of any carer you have to carry on caring, if appropriate (see carer's section for more information on carers' rights).

Note: Disabled young people leaving full time education also have a right for their needs to be assessed.

Step two: deciding if you are eligible for help

The local authority then decides whether or not it should provide or arrange community care services for you under its eligibility criteria.

Eligibility criteria are locally set rules on what type of needs the local authority will meet. Each authority sets its own eligibility criteria but these should comply with national guidance (called Fair Access to Care Services in England). Most local authorities have restricted who they provide support to and only provide support to people with 'critical' or 'substantial' needs (the other two categories are 'moderate' and 'low' needs). You can get more information about what these categories mean from RADAR.

Once your local authority has decided that you have eligible needs it is obliged to provide you with support.

Step three: care and support planning

Once the local authority has decided that it should provide or arrange help for you it should then **draw up a care plan**. This should say what your needs are and what services you will receive. You should be provided with a copy of the written record of the care plan.

You should be offered the chance of having direct payments – cash payments so you can buy and manage your own support – instead of services directly arranged by social services. It's not just disabled adults who can opt for direct payments, parents of disabled children have a right to them too.

Direct payments are for support at home and in the community – you can't use them to pay for care home accommodation, although you can use them for short breaks if you choose.

You can have a combination of direct payments and direct service provision from your local authority if you like.

If you opt for direct payments and need to employ a personal assistant or support worker, you should be referred to a direct payments support service which can advise and support you and provide you with a full pay-roll service. If that sounds daunting, it isn't if you get the right support. If you don't fancy managing the money yourself, another option is enlisting support of family and friends or an organisation you really trust and setting up a system for them to manage the money for you.

You can't usually employ a close family member as a support worker unless it's the best way of meeting your needs.

The National Centre for Independent Living has details of local support services (see details below). Plus an organisation called "In Control" has more information about all the different ways you can take more control over your support arrangements. See below for an explanation of 'individual budgets' which increasing numbers of local authorities across the UK are moving towards and proposals for a 'right to control'.

Step four: financial assessment and charging

Having decided it should arrange or provide services for you or give you direct payments, the local authority will carry out a financial assessment to work out how much you should contribute towards the cost of those services. Local authorities are not obliged to charge people (unless it's for residential care) but the vast majority, sadly, do. There is government guidance on this (and there are slightly different rules in each nation in the UK) but every area implements it differently and how much you contribute really depends on where you live. Do get a copy of your local authority's charging policy.

When the financial assessment is carried out your local authority should check whether you are getting all the benefits you are entitled to. Certain types of income are sacrosanct and cannot be taken into account. This includes any earnings from work (in Scotland unfortunately earnings are not exempt) and the mobility component of Disabled Living Allowance. They will need to work out what your disability related expenditure is and make sure they leave you enough to live on.

If you get a direct payment, your local authority may either take off an element for your contribution before they pay it to you or give you the full amount and then ask you pay the charge.

A service cannot be taken away from someone who cannot or does not pay, although the local authority can seek to recover money owed through court action.

Step five: providing support and reviewing your needs

Key things to note:

> ❯ You will be given a 'care manager' who is responsible for organising your support services and liaising with other agencies you need support from.

> ❯ If the local authority is arranging your support services, it will increasingly be provided by private or voluntary sector agencies rather than by the council itself. Social care providers have to register with the relevant inspection and regulation body (see below).

> ❯ Once your support is in place, the local authority should check it's working for you and review your needs after 3 months and annually thereafter. If your needs change or a carer leaves, you can ask for a review.

> ❯ There has been a gradual cutting back in the help local authorities provide in recent years. However you cannot have your support withdrawn – e.g. if they change their eligibility criteria – without first being reassessed.

If you are not happy with the service you get

If you are refused an assessment, denied support services or direct payments, if you are made to wait an age before support is put in place or if you are unhappy about any other aspect of the way your local authority has dealt with you then you can make a complaint. Each local authority has to have a complaints procedure and has to tell you about how to make a complaint. If that doesn't resolve the issue you can also complain to the local authority Monitoring Officer (usually the Chief Executive) who is responsible for ensuring the authority acts lawfully and fairly. If you exhaust the complaints procedure you can take your problem to the Ombudsman (Local Government Ombudsman – England; Scottish Public Services Ombudsman; Public Service Ombudsman for Wales or the Northern Ireland Ombudsman). Or you could consider bringing legal action – a judicial review, but you would need to take legal advice about this and seek legal representation. It will be well worth getting advice from a local Centre for Independent Living, local disability association or national disability organisation to check your rights and see if they can advocate for you. Your local councillor and local MP are also worth approaching for help.

For complaints about social care providers (whether home-based care providers or residential care) you can notify the relevant inspection agency (see below – there are different ones for each nation). In England they don't investigate individual cases but they will take it into account in deciding whether the provider is meeting the minimum standards of care they are supposed to provide. In Scotland and Wales the regulator may investigate your complaint.

Social care – differences across the nations

The system described above broadly applies across all four nations of the UK even though social care is one of the key responsibilities that has been devolved from Westminster Government to national governments. Much of the legislation is very similar but national guidance varies. Key differences are that

In Scotland:-

❯ Personal care is free for people over 65. That covers things like help with dressing, using a hoist, bathing, continence management, simple treatments, counselling and help to prepare food.

❯ Earnings are taken into account in financial assessments for social care.

❯ In Scotland there is a right to support and treatment for mental health problems, unlike in the rest of the UK.

In Northern Ireland:-

❯ Health and social care are provided by health and social care trusts, commissioned by 4 joint Health and Social Care Boards

❯ If you are over 75 you are not charged for your home help service.

Extra help for people with high support needs

The Independent Living Funds were established to give cash to disabled people with high support needs to live at home. To get help, new applicants must:

❯ receive services or cash to the value of at least £320 per week from their local authority (£200 in Northern Ireland)

❯ be at least 16 and under 65 years of age;

❯ receive the highest rate care component of the Disability Living Allowance

❯ have savings of less than £18,500.

❯ have a care package which won't cost more than £785 a week in total (including the ILF contribution)

If you think you may be eligible, ask your local authority social services to support your application.

Independent Living Funds
PO Box 7525, Nottingham NG2 4ZT.
☎ 0845 601 8815. @ funds@ilf.org.uk ⓦ www.ilf.org.uk

Choosing the right support and services for you

Even if your needs are too low to qualify for social service support, or you have to pay
for your own care, your local authority should be able to give you information and guidance about the kinds of services that would help you. These may be from the private sector, voluntary organisations or charities. The different country inspection agencies can also provide information on choosing services and access to inspection reports on different providers.

www.papool.co.uk is a browsable website of Personal Assistants and PA users, with information about each person and who or what they are looking for. Members can search the database whether they are recruiting or looking for work. The site has an e-mail facility so that personal details do not have to be revealed until the time is right and members are rated by recommendation to give reassurance. PA Pool was designed by an experienced PA user.

In Control is developing a web-based resource called 'Shop4Support' where you will be able to choose and buy a wide range of services.

Long-term/ continuing health care

The NHS also has responsibilities to meet people's needs for services like physiotherapy, speech and language therapy, rehabilitation services (for example low vision or mobility training for blind and partially sighted people, rehabilitation for people who have
had strokes).

The NHS is responsible for providing long-term or continuing health care (whatever setting that's provided in – at home, in residential or nursing care) and there are criteria governing who is eligible for such support. Age Concern produces a helpful factsheet: "NHS continuing healthcare, NHS-funded nursing care and intermediate care".

If your needs are deemed to be primarily 'medical' then they are the responsibility of the health service, rather than social services. NHS care is free, whereas social care is means tested. Primary Care Trusts and Local Health Boards have powers to pool funding with social services so people's needs can be met more seamlessly. However this doesn't happen routinely. People have problems when they have been receiving direct payments for social care but are then told their needs are such that health will be taking over responsibility. There is no 'right' to direct payments for health care, although this is going to be piloted. However in the best authorities, PCTs/Local health boards will agree to transfer funding to social services so people can continue to exercise control over their support services.

The future: a right to control

All local authorities in England are supposed to be moving towards a system of self-directed support and individual budgets in which disabled people are supported to determine their own needs and support plan, drawing on a range of funding sources and with real choice and control over how support is provided. This builds on direct payments but 'individual budgets' will involve people being told up front what resources are at their disposal and having greater flexibility over what they spend the money on and how it is managed. The Government is taking powers in the Welfare Reform Bill to create a 'right to control' for disabled adults in Britain over a wide range of public service support: employment support, educational support, Disabled Facilities Grants, Access to Work funding and social care. The 'right to control' will be piloted first to test how different funding streams can be brought together so disabled people can have an individual budget covering all of them.

National Centre for Independent Living (NCIL)
4th Floor, Hampton House, 20 Albert Embankment, London SE1 7TJ.
☎ 020 7587 1663. Textphone: 020 7587 1177. @ ncil@ncil.org.uk
Ⓦ www.ncil.org.uk

NCIL is a national membership organisation run and controlled by disabled people and funded to work in England. Its aim is that all disabled people have choice and control over all aspects of their lives with support when needed. It promotes the use of direct payments as a way of achieving independent living. It provides information and carries out research, training and consultancy and policy development with government in relation to personal assistance and Independent Living. It produces a range of publications and organises networking meetings to share experiences nationally and regionally. It also provides a link between people seeking work as personal assistants and those wanting to employ them.

In Control

Swan Courtyard, Coventry Road,
Birmingham B26 1BU.
☎ 0121 708 3031.
@ admin@in-control.org.uk
Ⓦ www.in-control.org.uk

In Control is a social enterprise whose mission is to help create a new welfare system in which everyone is in control of their lives as full citizens. They have worked with disabled people and local authorities to design a new system for care and support- Self-Directed Support. The Government now wants all local authorities to change their systems to Self-Directed Support. A wealth of information on how self-directed support works is available from their website.

United Kingdom Home Care Association

Group House, 2nd Floor, 52 Sutton Court Road, Sutton SM1 4SL.
☎ 020 8288 5291.
@ helpline@ukhca.co.uk
Ⓦ www.ukhca.co.uk

UKHCA represents and supports home care agencies and operates a code of practice for its members, a list of whom can be supplied or found on its website.

Inspection & Registration Bodies

Care Quality Commission

7th Floor, New Kings Beam House,
22 Upper Ground, London SE1 9BW.

☎ 03000 616161
Ⓦ www.cqc.org.uk

Department of Health, Social Services & Public Safety

Castle Buildings, Stormont,
Belfast BT4 3SJ.
☎ 028 9052 0500.
@ ssi@dhsspsni.gov.uk
Ⓦ www.dhsspsni.gov.uk

Scottish Commission for the Regulation of Care

Compass House, 11 Riverside Drive,
Dundee DD1 4NY.
☎ 01382 207100.
@ enquiries@carecommission.com
Ⓦ www.carecommission.com

Care & Social Services Inspectorate Wales

4-5, Charnwood Court, Heol Billingsley,
Parc Nantgarw, Nantgarw, Cardiff
CF15 7QZ.
☎ 01443 848450.
@ cssiw@wales.gsi.gov.uk
Ⓦ www.cssiw.org.uk

LEGAL AND CONSUMER SERVICES

Legal Advice

Most people need to make use of legal services at some time, whether for personal family matters or to follow up a matter of law in relation to disability discrimination or claims for disability related benefits such as Disability Living Allowance or Attendance Allowance. People can be put off seeking legal advice because of real or perceived problems of access and cost. Remember that legally qualified professionals are providing a service and must comply with the Disability Discrimination Acts, whether their service is charged for or provided at no cost. You should expect an accessible service and demand reasonable adjustments if they are not already in place. Remember also that some legal services do not charge for their services – examples of these organisations include Law Centres, the bar's Pro Bono Unit and Citizens advice Bureaux.

Community Legal Advice
☎ 0845 345 4345.
Ⓦ www.clsdirect.org.uk

Community Legal Advice is the Government agency responsible for helping people get legal help in non-criminal matters. It provides free advice by phone on a wide range of matters for those who qualify for legal aid. It can also put you in touch with your nearest face-to-face advice provider. The CLA site provides particularly helpful advice and leaflets about discrimination law and segments its advice by type – disability, age, gender, race, etc. CLA covers England and Wales.

For other parts of the UK contact:

Northern Ireland Legal Services Commission.
☎ 028 9040 8888.
Ⓦ www.nilsc.org.uk

Scottish Legal Aid Board.
☎ 0845 122 8686.
Ⓦ www.slab.org.uk

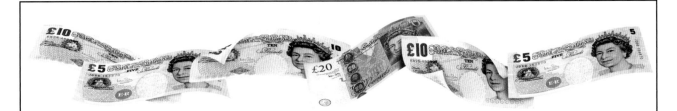
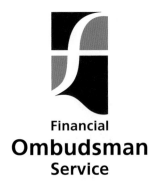

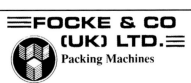
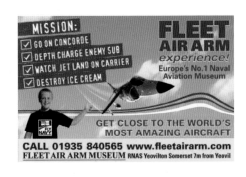

The Children's Legal Centre
University of Essex, Wivenhoe Park,
Colchester CO4 3SQ.
☎ 01206 872466. @ clc@essex.ac.uk
Ⓦ www.childrenslegalcentre.com

The CLC is a national charity concerned with law and policy affecting children and young people. It offers a free, confidential service from telephone advice through to full legal representation. The website contains information on many aspects of the law for young people, parents and carers in a user-friendly format.

Citizens Advice Bureaux (CAB)
You will find a CAB in most towns in England and Wales. The Citizens Advice web sites can tell you where your nearest Bureau is located.
Ⓦ **www.citizensadvice.org.uk** and **www. adviceguide.org.uk (www.cas.org.uk** for Scotland and **www.citizensadvice.co.uk** for Northern Ireland)

The Citizens Advice service helps people resolve their legal, money and other problems by providing free information and advice from over 3,200 locations, and by influencing policymakers. The majority of CAB advisers are trained volunteers, helping people to resolve over 5.5 million problems every year. All Citizens Advice Bureaux in England, Wales and Northern Ireland are members of Citizens Advice, the national charity which sets standards for advice and equal opportunities and supports bureaux with an information system, training and other services.

Disability Law Service
39-45 Cavell Street, London E1 2BP.
☎ 020 7791 9800.
Typetalk: 18001 020 7791 9800.
@ advice@dls.org.uk
Ⓦ www.dls.org.uk

The Disability Law Service is a charity providing free and confidential legal advice, information and case-work services to disabled people, their families, carers and advocates. It provides specialist advice on Consumer matters, Community Care, Disability Discrimination, Employment, Further and Higher Education and Welfare Benefits (Greater London area). The DLS National Advice Line can provide access to a lawyer or qualified legal advisor. DLS caseworkers will assist the individual to seek help elsewhere if they cannot take on the case themselves. A comprehensive range of factsheets on all the areas of law covered is produced.

The Independent Panel for Special Education Advice (IPSEA)
6 Carlow Mews, Woodbridge,
Suffolk IP12 1EA.
☎ 0800 0184016.
Ⓦ www.ipsea.org.uk

IPSEA gives free and independent education related legal advice and support in England and Wales through Helplines, written information on their website and in print, advice, support and representation (when needed) in appeals to the Special Educational Needs and Disability Tribunal and disability discrimination advice and training in collaboration with the Equality and Human Rights Commission.

Law Centres Federation
293-299 Kentish Town Road,
London NW5 2TJ.
☎ 020 7428 4400.
Ⓦ www.lawcentres.org.uk

The LCF does not itself provide legal advice but can provide information about Law Centres to people living or working in their catchment areas.

The Solicitors Room
☎ 01925 422942.
Ⓦ www.thesolicitorsroom.com

If visiting a solicitor is a problem, then The SolicitorsRoom.com may provide a solution. This organisation, set up in association with the Disability Alliance, provides an on-line service whereby a disabled person can be put in touch with a solicitor who meets their requirements in respect of the type of work to be carried out and geographical proximity. A computer programme has been developed so that documents can be transferred and seen at any time without the security disadvantages of email. There is no charge to register with the service although subsequent legal fees will be agreed with the solicitor.

Consumer Matters

Disabled people have the right not to be discriminated against in the provision of goods or services (see Discrimination section), but beyond this may also call on the wider protection of consumer rights legislation. For example, buying products from home, whether by mail order, on the internet or at the door, may be more convenient than getting to the shops but it can also change the relationship between buyer and seller so there are a number of safeguards such as cooling off periods.

Local authority trading standards officers can take action against dishonest traders, but this will often be too late for those who have been victims of their scams. However, advice and information to consumers is available from a number of sources:

Consumer Direct
☎ 0845 404 0506.
Textphone: 0845 128 1384.
Ⓦ www.consumerdirect.gov.uk

Consumer Direct provides information and advice on consumer issues by telephone and on its website. It works in association with local authority Trading Standards services. Consumer Direct cannot take action against a trader, although it can advise on how to do so and refer enquirers to other bodies that can assist. The website includes advice on how to avoid scams and find trustworthy traders.

Consumer Focus
4th Floor, Artillery House, Artillery Row, London SW1P 1RT
☎ 020 7799 7900.
Ⓦ www.consumerfocus.org.uk

Consumer Focus is the new body which campaigns for a fair deal for customers. It was created through the merger of energywatch, Postwatch and the National Consumer Council. Consumer Focus has the right to investigate any consumer complaint if it's of wider interest and the ability to make an official super-complaint about failing services. However, it can't provide advice.

Elsewhere in the UK contact:

Consumer Focus Scotland
Royal Exchange House, 100 Queen Street, Glasgow G1 3DN
☎ 0141 226 5261

Consumer Focus Wales
3rd Floor, Capital Tower, Greyfriars Road, Cardiff CF10 3AG
☎ 02920 787100

Consumer Focus Post - Northern Ireland
4th Floor, 24-26 Arthur Street, Belfast BT1 4GF
☎ 028 9027 9300

Office of Fair Trading
Fleetbank House, 2-6 Salisbury Square, London EC4Y 8JX.
☎ 08457 224499.
ⓦ www.oft.gov.uk

The OFT is the UK's consumer and competition authority. It is not able to deal with individual enquiries but sponsors Consumer Direct and issues a wide range of publications and leaflets.

Utilities

Utility companies are required to provide services to meet the specific needs of disabled customers. This may include special arrangements for meter reading, providing bills and other material in alternative formats and giving priority and other support if there is a stoppage or breakdown in supplies. If you feel you may need help in any way contact the companies involved and ask to be placed on their priority list. This can often mean a faster reconnection when you experience, for example, a power cut or help collecting water if you get cut off.

Complaints concerning energy and postal companies should be directed to Consumer Direct.

Many utility companies have established Trust Funds that make grants to people struggling with utility and other household debts. The actual terms of the grants vary, some are only for customers while others may be for anyone living in the company's area, and may require applications to be supported by a Social Worker or advice worker. Several of these trusts are managed by Charis. Details of which trusts and links to the relevant trust website are provided from its own website: www.charisgrants.com

Energy

Ofgem
9 Millbank, London SW1P 3GE.
☎ 020 7901 7000.
ⓦ www.ofgem.gov.uk

Ofgem (the Office of Gas & Electricity Markets) is the regulator of the gas and electricity industries. It does not deal with individual consumer complaints.

In Northern Ireland a similar role is carried out by Ofreg,
☎ 028 9031 1575. ⓦ ofreg.nics.gov.uk

Energy Supply Ombudsman
PO Box 966, Warrington WA4 9DF.
☎ 0845 055 0760.
Textphone: 0845 051 1513.
ⓦ www.energy-ombudsman.org.uk

The Energy Supply Ombudsman decides what action should be taken when a customer and energy supplier can't agree over a complaint.

Telecommunications

Ofcom

Riverside House, 2A Southwark Bridge Road, London SE1 9HA.
☎ 020 7981 3040.
Textphone: 020 7981 3043.
ⓦ www.ofcom.org.uk

Ofcom is the regulatory body covering both telecommunications and broadcasting and also acts as the consumer body for most of the industry.

OTELO (Office of the Telecommunications Ombudsmam)

PO Box 730, Warrington WA4 6WU.
☎ 0845 050 1614.
Textphone: 0845 051 1513.
@ enquiries@otelo.org.uk
ⓦ www.otelo.org.uk

Water

Ofwat

City Centre Tower, 7 Hill Street, Birmingham B5 4UA.
☎ 0121 625 1300.
ⓦ www.ofwat.gov.uk

Ofwat is the regulator of companies providing water and sewerage services in England and Wales. It establishes minimum standards for the companies involved and monitors their performance.

In Scotland a similar regulatory role is carried out by the Water Industry Commission for Scotland, Ochil House, Springkerse Business Park, Stirling FK7 7XE.
☎ 01786 430200.
ⓦ www.watercommission.co.uk

Consumer Council for Water

Victoria Square House, Victoria Square, Birmingham B2 4AJ.
☎ 0845 039 2837.
Textphone: 0121 345 1044.
ⓦ www.ccwater.org.uk

CC Water represents the interests of consumers of water and sewerage services in England and Wales. It can take up unresolved complaints that consumers have with their supply companies.

In Scotland a similar service is offered by Waterwatch Scotland, Forrester Lodge, Inglewood, Alloa FK10 2HU.
@ info@waterwatchscotland.org
ⓦ www.waterwatchscotland.org

WaterSure allows some customers with water meters to use extra water without worrying about getting a high bill. To be eligible, customers must be receiving income related benefits and either have 3 or more children at home or a medical condition that requires extra water. These customers can have their water bill capped at the amount of the average household bill for their water company. Information can be provided by CC Water.

LEISURE ACTIVITIES

The whole range of leisure activities is available to disabled people according to their tastes, interests and inclinations. In most instances people can continue with those that they took part in before they were disabled, perhaps with some adapted equipment or support. A local library is a good place to get information about leisure activities and organisations in an area and a local disability organisation may be able to put you in touch with special interest organisations.

Arts

A wide range of organisations related to the arts are available whether you want to participate or just appreciate.

The Arts Council of England
14 Great Peter Street, London
SW1P 3NQ.
☎ 0845 300 6200.
Textphone: 020 7973 6564.
✉ enquiries@artscouncil.org.uk
🌐 www.artscouncil.org.uk

The Arts Council of England is responsible for arts funding and development in England and also provides information and advice to artists and arts organisations.

Elsewhere in UK contact:

The Arts Council of Northern Ireland
77 Malone Road, Belfast BT9 6AQ
☎ 028 9038 5200.
🌐 www.artscouncil-ni.org

The Scottish Arts Council
12 Manor Place, Edinburgh EH3 7DD.
☎ 0131 226 6051.
🌐 www.scottisharts.org.uk

The Arts Council of Wales
9 Museum Place, Cardiff CF1 3NX.
☎ 029 2037 6500.
Textphone: 029 2039 0027.
🌐 www.artswales.org

Disability Cultural Projects
🌐 www.disabilityarts.info

DCP produces a weekly electronic newsletter of opportunities, an events list and has developed an evolving online arts access guide – artsaccessuk.org. The website also contains extensive links to disability arts organisations and archived material from the National Disability Arts Forum that closed in 2008.

Theatre Resource aims to advance and promote creativity, culture and heritage of disabled people and other socially excluded groups in Essex and Hertfordshire. It arranges a wide range of programmes and events. Contact Theatre Resource, High Street, Chipping Ongar, Essex CM5 0AD. ☎ 01277 365626. Textphone: 01277 365003
W www.theatre-resource.org.uk

MAGIC Deaf Arts is a grouping of 16 of the major museums and art galleries in London. Each provides events and facilities for deaf and hard of hearing visitors, including specialist tours and employing sign interpreters at public talks and lectures. A calendar of events is available on www.magicdeaf.org.uk

Artsline

c/o 21 Pine Court, Wood Lodge Gardens, Bromley BR1 2WA.
☎/Textphone: 020 7388 2227.
@ access@artsline.org.uk
W www.artsline.org.uk

Artsline provides free online and telephone information services for disabled people on arts and leisure events and activities in and around London. Full details provided on access and provision for disabl2ed people at London arts and entertainment venues.

National Theatre

South Bank, London SE1 9PX
☎ 020 7452 3000.
@ access@nationaltheatre.org.uk
W www.nationaltheatre.org.uk

The National Theatre aims to be accessible and welcoming to all. Its three auditoriums have allocated wheelchair spaces and assistance dogs are welcome. For deaf and hearing impaired it provides audio-described performances and synopses notes on CD. For blind and visually-impaired it provides captioned performances, touch tours and Braille cast lists. Its access mailing list offers free information on CD, in Braille and large print via email.

Music and the Deaf

The Media Centre, 7 Northumberland Street, Huddersfield HD1 1RL.
☎ 01484 483115.
Textphone: 01484 483117.
W www.matd.org.uk

Music and the Deaf helps deaf people of all ages access music and the performing arts. It provides talks, signed theatre performances and workshops. In West Yorkshire it runs after-school clubs, a Deaf Youth Orchestra and has developed programmes and guidance to deliver the music national curriculum to deaf children. Music and the Deaf also runs training days and collaborative projects with orchestras, opera, theatre and dance companies.

Shape

LVS Resource Centre, 356 Holloway Road, London N7 6PA.
☎ 020 7619 6160.
Textphone; 020 7619 6161.
W www.shapearts.org.uk

Shape offers a range of activities to enable disabled and deaf people to participate and enjoy arts and cultural activities in London. Shape Tickets is a service offering its members tickets, often at reduced prices, at venues throughout London coupled with access assistance and transport if required.

Signed Performances In Theatre

6 Thirlmere Drive, Lymm, Cheshire
WA13 9PE.
☎ 01925 754231.
Textphone: 01925 757115.
Ⓦ www.spit.org.uk

SPIT promotes BSL interpreted performances in the mainstream theatre and provides a link between arts organisations and the Deaf community. Its website includes a searchable directory of signed and captioned performances nationwide.

STAGETEXT

1st Floor, 54 Commercial Street,
London E1 6LT.
☎ 020 7377 0540.
Textphone: 020 7247 7801.
@ enquiries@stagetext.org
Ⓦ www.stagetext.org

STAGETEXT provides access to the theatre for deaf, deafened and hard of hearing people through captioning. The full text, together with character names, sound effects and off-stage noises, is shown on LED displays as the words are spoken or sung. Around 200 productions are captioned each year in over 80 venues across the UK. Information on forthcoming performances is given on its website.

Vocaleyes

1st Floor, 54 Commercial Street,
London E1 6LT.
☎ 020 7375 1043.
@ enquiries@vocaleyes.co.uk
Ⓦ www.vocaleyes.co.uk

National organisation established to provide audio description for performances in the theatre and now also works in museums, galleries and architectural heritage sites. It has provided over 600 performances at more than 100 venues to date. A programme of its forthcoming events is published in print, Braille and on tape as well as on their website

Cinemas

In the past few cinemas were accessible to people with impaired mobility, hearing or sight. The widescale development of new cinema buildings over the last 10 years or so began to change that in respect to physical access, with at least some screens in multiplexes having spaces for wheelchair users.

Now a programme is underway to substantially increase both the number of cinemas equipped to show films with digital sub-titles and audio description and the number of films that are available. A website has been developed to give information on subtitled and audio described films and where they are being shown – www.yourlocalcinema.com

The Cinema Exhibitors' Association has a national card for disabled people that verifies that they are entitles to a free ticket for a person accompanying them to the cinema. To qualify applicants must receive the disability living allowance or attendance allowance or be a registered blind person. A £5.50 administration charge is made and the card is valid for 3 years. Application forms can be obtained from participating cinemas or downloaded from the website. Contact The Card Network, Network House, St Ives Way, Sandycroft CH5 2QS. ☎ 0845 123 1295. Textphone: 0845 123 1297.   @ info@ceacard.co.uk Ⓦ www.ceacard.co.uk

Sport

There are a multitude of organisations concerned with sporting provision for disabled people – they may be local or national, concerned with a single sport or many, catering solely for disabled people or involved with inclusive services. Specialist organisations often have an important role in both introducing people to sport and for those wishing to be involved in competitions. "Taster" sessions, which give the opportunity to try a range of activities, are often arranged locally at local sports or leisure centrest. For information on facilities and sporting groups in your local area contact the local authority Sports Development Officer or the following organisations may be able to point you in the right direction.

www.activeplaces.com is a database giving information on sports facilities in England. Information includes contact details, activities available, charges (if any), whether membership is required and information on accessibility for disabled people. The database, is being expanded to include as many venues as possible, both public and private, and currently has over 50,000 entries.

English Federation of Disability Sport
Manchester Metropolitan University, Alsager Campus, Hassall Road, Alsager, Stoke on Trent ST7 2HL. ☎ 0161 247 5294. Textphone: 0161 247 5644.
Ⓦ federation@efds.co.uk   Ⓦ www.efds.co.uk

EFDS is an umbrella group of disability sports organisations which acts as a united voice influencing policy makers and the mainstream Governing Bodies of sports to develop opportunities for disabled people to become more involved as competitors, recreational participants, administrators, officials and coaches. It also seeks to create greater co-operation between disability sports organisations and works with the following National Disability Sports Organisations that are recognized by Sport England:

BALASA
Special Olympics
CP Sport
Dwarf Athletics
British Blind Sport
Wheelpower – British Wheelchair Support

For other parts of the UK contact:

Disability Sport Northern Ireland

Adelaide House, Falcon Road, Belfast BT12 6RD.
☎ 028 9038 7062.
Ⓦ www.dsni.co.uk

Scottish Disability Sport

Caledonia House, South Gyle, Edinburgh EH12 9DQ.
☎ 0131 317 1130.
Ⓦ www.scottishdisabilitysport.com

Disability Sport Wales

Welsh Institute of Sport, Sophia Gardens, Cardiff CF11 9SW.
☎ 0845 846 0021.
Ⓦ www.disabilitysportwales.org

In some areas local organisations have been formed to provide a range of sporting and sometimes other recreational activities for disabled people. These may use premises owned by the local council or other bodies but a number have their own purpose-built Centres.

> OXSRAD – the Integrated Sports Centre (the Oxford Sport and Recreation Association for Disabled People) is an integrated Sport and Leisure Centre on the outskirts of Oxford. It offers an Inclusive Fitness Suite, sports and activity halls, a spa bath, treatment room and a bar. Activities include bdminton, archery, snooker and pool, indoor bowls, table-tennis and disabled trampolining. There is also the opportunity to participate in art, music and dance classes. The centre hosts an integrated youth club each week and a programme for school-aged children during the summer holidays. OXSRAD is based at Court Place Farm, Marsh Lane, Marston, Oxford OX3 0NQ. ☎ 01865 741336.
> Ⓦ www.oxsrad.org

The following are some of the organisations and projects concerned with helping disabled people take part in specific sporting activities.

British Disabled Angling Association

9 Yew Tree Road, Delves, Walsall WS5 4NQ.
☎ 01922 860912 (answerphone). Ⓦ www.bdaa.co.uk

BDDA represents all disabled anglers across UK, including coarse, sea, specimen and game fishing. Services include:

Specialised angling courses
Group development
Access audits of fishing areas
Training people to coach disabled people
Disability awareness training.

NDCS Deaf Friendly Football Club Project is a 3-year project run by the National Deaf Children's Society to remove the barriers faced by many deaf children and young people to participating in football. The project will work at all levels of the game through the development of information and resources, the provision of training and setting up a youth deaf football infrastructure in England. For information contact Deaf Friendly Football Club project, NDCS, 15 Dufferin Street, London EC1Y 8UR. SMS 07966 341 022.

@ hayley.brown@ndcs.org.uk or see www.ndcs.org

The Inclusive Fitness Initiative

MLS Ltd, 4 Park Square, Newton Chambers Road, Thorncliffe Park, Chapeltown, Sheffield S35 2PH.
☎ 0114 257 2060.
@ info@inclusivefitness.org
Ⓦ www.inclusivefitness.org

The IFA, originally launched by the English Federation for Disability Sport, promotes the provision and management of integrated facilities for disabled people in general fitness centres. It accredits venues that provide accessible facilities, inclusive fitness equipment, appropriate staff straining and inclusive marketing.

Wheels for All

Cycling Projects, 1 Enterprise Park, Shearer Way, Pendlebury, Manchester M27 8WA.
☎ 0161 745 9944.
Ⓦ www.cycling.org.uk

Wheels for All operates centres from which a range of cycles with adaptations for disabled people can be borrowed or hired. Some of these centres are based at sports centres or urban parks while others provide the opportunity to use routes in country areas. Sixteen Wheels for All Centres currently exist with more in the pipeline.

Spectator Sports

The creation of new and enlarged arenas, the greater awareness of the needs of disabled people and the impact of the Disability Discrimination Act and other regulations has lead to improved facilities for disabled spectators in many places. However, limitations remain. Some arise from the nature of the feature provided, such as a commentary for visually impaired spectators at a football match or a raised viewing platform for wheelchair users at a racecourse, while others result from lack of provision. In some cases, such as golf tournaments, spectator arrangements are for a particular event. Any disabled person needing any particular facility or service or needing to know its location within a ground is still recommended to contact the venue in advance.

Association of Wheelchair & Ambulant Disabled Supporters

c/o 2 Coopers Fold, Ribbleton, Preston PR2 6HW.
☎ 01772 700788
Ⓦ www.awads.co.uk

The AWADS website contains access information on League and many non-league football grounds in England and Scotland. Many of the entries also include members' comments.

National Association of Disabled Spectators

PO Box 2909, Reading, RG1 9DL.
☎ 0845 230 6237.
@ info@nads.org.uk
Ⓦ www.nads.org.uk

NADS was established to work for good facilities for disabled spectators at football grounds. It now has links with Disabled Supporters Associations at many clubs and its website includes information on facilities for disabled fans at grounds around the country.

Leisure Adult Education

Although much adult or continuing education is directed at vocational subjects leading to enhanced employment opportunities, many people want to learn more about a subject for their own personal interest.

Day or evening courses are offered in specialist adult education centres, schools, colleges or other community premises. There are examples of courses being organized specifically for disabled students but it is increasingly possible for disabled people to participate in mainstream courses. Most brochures or prospectuses give general information for disabled people and the name of a contact in the institution. Most adult education courses are organised by Adult Education Colleges but there are a variety of other providers including University Extra Mural Departments.

Workers' Educational Association

65 Clifton Street, London EC2A 4JE.
☎ 020 7375 3092.
@ national@wea.org.uk
Ⓦ www.wea.org.uk

WEA Northern Ireland

1 Fitzwilliam Street, Belfast BT9 6AW.
☎ 028 9032 9718.
@ info@wea-ni.com
Ⓦ www.wea-ni.com

WEA Scottish Association

Riddles Court, 322 Lawnmarket, Edinburgh EH1 2PG.
☎ 0131 226 3456.
@ hq@weascotland.org.uk

WEA South Wales

7 Coopers Yard, Curren Road, Cardiff CF10 5NB.
☎ 029 2023 5277.
Ⓦ www.swales.wea.org.uk

WEA Coleg Harlech

Harlech, Gwynedd LL46 2PU.
☎ 01766 781900.
Ⓦ www.harlech.ac.uk

The WEA is a major national voluntary adult education organisation providing over 10,000 courses a year. These are mainly arranged through local branches.

University of the Third Age

The Third Age Trust, 19 East Street, Bromley BR1 1QH.
☎ 020 8466 6139.
Ⓦ www.u3a.org.uk

U3A promotes learning by people no longer in full-time employment through autonomous local learning groups. There are around 500 independent local U3A groups in the UK with around 125,000 members in total.

Residential Course Centres

Many people find it helpful to learn or develop a skill or leisure interest on a short residential course. This may be for practical reasons such as the difficulty of getting to a series of day or evening classes. However, others find sharing an interest with others over a period of several days enriches the whole experience.

Adult Residential Colleges Association – ARCA

6 Bath Road, Felixstowe IP11 7JW.

@ arcasec@aol.com ⓦ www.arca.uk.net

The ARCA colleges specialise in short-stay residential adult education courses for the general public. Each college has its own programme of weekend, midweek and day courses, and some offer summer schools and courses leading to recognised qualifications. Accommodation ranges upwards from the simply comfortable. Many of the colleges have accommodation and facilities for people with disabilities although individual requirements should be checked before booking.

Days Out

While most modern tourist attractions should be able to cater for disabled visitors it is advisable to check in advance if you have any specific requirements, if the attraction is large or for particular events.

Sites with a conservation aim, including historic buildings, nature reserves, forests, industrial heritage displays etc, can have particular limitations for disabled visitors. Several organisations with a number of such sites open to the public have worked to improve facilities for their disabled visitors. The following have specialist publications and web pages on their facilities:

CADW: Welsh Historic Monuments

Plas Carew, Unit 5/7 Cefn Coed, Park Nantgarw, Cardiff CF15 7QQ.

☎ 01443 336000. @ cadw@wales.gsi. gov.uk ⓦ www.cadw.wales.gov.uk

Historic Scotland

Longmore House, Salisbury Place, Edinburgh EH9 1SH.

☎ 0131 668 8800.

ⓦ www.historic-scotland.gov.uk

English Heritage

Customer Services Department, PO Box 567, Swindon SN2 2YP.

☎ 0870 333 1182.

Textphone: 01793 414878.

@ customers@english-heritage.org.uk

ⓦ www.english-heritage.org.uk

The National Trust

Membership Department, PO Box 39, Warrington WA5 7WD.

☎ 0844 800 1895.

Textphone: 0844 800 4410.

@ accessforall@nationaltrust.org.uk

Ⓦ www.nationaltrust.org.uk

National Trust for Scotland

Weymss House. 28 Charlotte Square, EH2 4ET.

☎ 0131 243 9300.   Ⓦ www.nts.org.uk

Royal Society for the Protection of Birds

The Lodge, Potton Road, Sandy SG19 2DL.

☎ 01767 680551.   Ⓦ www.rspb.org.uk

www.disabledgo.info provides on-line access guides to a number of towns and areas in the UK. These include detailed access information gathered by personal inspection at a wide range of entertainment venues, places to visit, catering establishments and shops.

Reading

Enjoying books can be difficult for a wide range of disabled people who, for whatever reason, cannot use printed matter. Audio books are increasingly available in libraries or bookshops. In addition, the following organisations offer services that may help.

Bag Books

1 Stewarts Court, 218-220 Stewarts Road. London SW8 4UB.

☎ 020 7627 0444.

@ office@bagbooks.org

Ⓦ www.bagbooks.org

Bagbooks produces multi-sensory story packs for people with profound learning disabilities. The packs were originally designed for children but there are now also titles suitable for teenagers and adults.

Calibre Audio Library

Aylesbury HP22 5XQ.

☎ 01296 432339.

@ enquiries@calibre.org.uk

Ⓦ www.calibre.org.uk

Calibre, a national charity, has a wide range of unabridged books on cassette or MP3 disc for adults and children who are visually impaired or cannot use books. These are lent to members who can order by post or on the internet.

ClearVision

Linden Lodge School, 61 Princes Way, London SW19 6JB.

☎ 020 8789 9575.

Ⓦ www.clearvisionproject.org

ClearVision provides mainstream children's books incorporating Braille, print and pictures that can be shared by visually impaired children and sighted children and adults. Over 13000 books are available. They are suitable for children learning Braille, or who may do so in the future, but not for partially sighted children learning to read print. Membership is free to families.

Isis Publishing Ltd

7 Centremead, Osney Mead, Oxford OX2 0ES.

☎ 01865 250333.

@ sales@isis-publishing.co.uk

Ⓦ www.isis-publishing.co.uk

Major audio publisher of unabridged titles in cassette, compact disc and other formats to direct and internet customers.

Listening Books
12 Lant Street, London SE1 1QH.
☎ 020 7407 9417.
@ membership@listening-books.org.uk
Ⓦ www.listening-books.org.uk

Listening Books offers an audio book service to people for whom holding a book, turning a page or reading in the usual way is not possible.

RNIB National Library Service
PO Box 173, Peterborough PE2 6WS.
☎ 0845 762 6843.
@ cservices@rnib.org.uk
Ⓦ www.rnib.org.uk

The library service of the RNIB aims to ensure that visually impaired people have the same access to library facilities as sighted people. It offers a lending service, with many titles now available in electronic form as well as the more traditional aural and tactile formats

Ulverscroft
The Green, Bradgate Road, Ansty, Leicester LE7 7FU.
☎ 0116 236 4325.
Ⓦ www.edisure.com

Ulverscroft is a long established publisher of large print books. It also distributes audio books from other publishers and has 6 regional showrooms.

Television

Television is going digital all over the UK and the traditional TV signal (analogue) will be switched off. But don't worry about losing your TV service. You'll be able to qualify for support to help you convert your TV to receive a digital signal. And digital services will offer you lots of new advantages.

Digital Television (DTV) is an advanced technology that enables broadcasters to offer television with better picture and sound quality. Other advantages include: greater choice of channels, electronic program guides, audio description and subtitling for people with visual and audio impairments and interactive video and data services.

The Digital TV Switchover is the process of converting the UK's terrestrial television system (analogue) to digital. It is a Government policy and it will mean that almost everyone will be able to receive digital TV through their TV aerial. Terrestrial services are being switched off in a rolling programme region by region up until 2012 and being replaced with free digital TV and radio services (Freeview).

To keep your TV service, you will need to convert your TV to digital before your area's switchover date. In order to help older and disabled people, who may face greater barriers in switching to digital TV, the Switchover Help Scheme was introduced. This scheme is run by the BBC under an agreement with the Government and helps eligible people to make the change to digital on one of their TV sets. People are eligible, if they are:

- ❯ aged 75 or over,

- ❯ residents in care homes,

- ❯ in receipt of (or could receive) Attendance or Constant Attendance Allowance, mobility supplement or Disability Living Allowance (DLA),

- ❯ registered blind or partially sighted with their local authority.

If you qualify, the Help Scheme will explain digital TV to you clearly and simply. It can help you choose and install any equipment you need in your home, and if necessary fit, a new dish or aerial and help you afterwards if you want to ask more questions.

The Help Scheme Switchover will cost £40, unless you get Pension Credit, Income Support or income-based Jobseeker's Allowance, in which case the help is free. The help will also be free if you are an adult who receives one of the benefits above and Child Benefit for an eligible child who lives at the same address.

For more information on the scheme, if you would like to know if you are eligible or to find out the date when your region is due to be switched over, contact the Switchover Help Scheme:

- ❯ by post: Freepost, Switchover Help Scheme

- ❯ Freephone: 0800 4085 900

- ❯ Textphone (minicom): 0800 4085 936

- ❯ E-mail: info@helpscheme.co.uk

- ❯ Website: www.helpscheme.co.uk

Help Scheme information is also available in large print, on coloured paper, in Easy Read, in Braille, on CD, DVD or video tape with British Sign Language and subtitles.

Shopping

While some people find going to the shops to be a chore, for many going shopping, or looking round the shops is a leisure activity. Many disabled people have found this made easier by the growth of purpose built shopping centres.

Shopmobility schemes provide wheelchairs and scooters for use in about 300 shopping and other areas throughout UK. Some schemes can provide children's

wheelchairs, escorts or special services for people visiting their area. A Directory giving details of the services offered by each is published each year and is available on its website. Contact National Federation of Shopmobility, PO Box 6641, Christchurch BH23 9DQ.
☎ 08456 442446.   @ info@shopmobilityuk.org   Ⓦ www.shopmobilityuk.org

Other Activities

It is almost impossible to think of any form of leisure activity that does not have an organisation attached to it and many have an organisation devoted to encouraging the participation of disabled people. The following are some that may be useful.

Disabled Photographers' Society

PO Box 85, Longfield, Kent DA3 9BA.
☎ 01454 317754.
@ secretary@disabledphotographers.co.uk
Ⓦ www.disabledphotographers.co.uk

The Disabled Photographers' Society provides information on adaptations that can be made to cameras and other photographic equipment and has access to engineers who can carry these out if required. It arranges an annual exhibition of members' work and organises occasional photographic holidays and other events. The DPS has close ties with mainstream photographic bodies.

Event Mobility Charitable Trust

8 Bayliss Road, Kemerton, Tewkesbury GL20 7JH.
☎ 01386 725391.
@ eventmobility@hotmail.co.uk
Ⓦ www.eventmobility.org.uk

Some events are problematic for disabled people to attend because they extend over a large area and/or the facilities for spectators are of a temporary nature. Event Mobility provides powered scooters and wheelchairs at a range of events including flower shows, agricultural and countryside shows, major golf championships and horse shows. Bookings have to be made in advance and a donation of £17 for scooters or £10 for manual wheelchairs is requested. A list of events at which the service will be available and other information can be obtained from the above address (please send a stamped addressed envelope) or on the website.

Motorsport Endeavour

123 Ealing Village, London W5 2EB.
☎ 020 8991 2358.
@ info@motorsportendeavour.com
Ⓦ www.motorsportendeavour.com

Motorsport Endeavour has been formed to run events involving disabled people in all forms of motorsport. A wide-ranging programme is planned, including rallys, karting and visits to motorsport venues. The club is open both to drivers and people wishing to take other roles including as navigators, marshals, timekeepers or, simply, spectators. It is also establishing links for disabled people who are seeking employment in the industry. The club was founded by people who, following disability, have continued an involvement in various forms of motorsport.

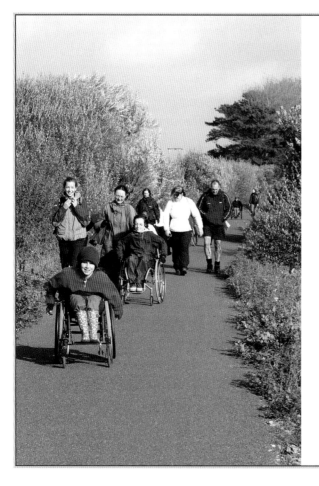

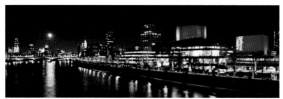

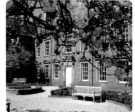

RNIB Recreation & Holidays

105 Judd Street, London WC1H 9NE.
☎ 020 7388 1266.
Ⓦ www.rnib.org

Information and advice on a wide range of leisure activities for visually impaired people is available from RNIB both for individuals who are thinking of taking up an activity and for providers. A number of publications are available.

RYA Sailability

RYA House, Ensign Way,
Hamble SO31 4YA.
☎ 0845 345 0493
@ sailability@rya.org.uk
Ⓦ www.rya.org.uk

Sailability promotes the participation of disabled people within the sailing community, whether as beginners through taster sessions and training or as competitors.

Thrive

The Geoffrey Udall Centre, Beech Hill,
Reading RG7 2AT.
☎ 0118 988 5688.
@ info@thrive.org.uk
Ⓦ www.thrive.org.uk

Thrive aims to improve the lives of elderly and disabled people through gardening and horticulture. It runs a number of demonstration gardens, supports a network of community or therapeutic gardening projects and has an extensive programme of training courses, many for people developing or running community gardening projects. Among Thrive's many publications are factsheets giving practical advice on a wide variety of topics. It also runs the Blind Gardeners' Club.

The www.carryongardening.co.uk website gives information of equipment and techniques to make gardening easier.

The Wheelyboat Trust

North Lodge, Burton Park, Petworth
GU28 0JT
☎ 01798 342222.
@ info@wheelyboats.org
Ⓦ www.wheelyboats.org

The Trust places specially designed Wheelyboats on lakes and other waters in all parts of the British Isles where they can be used for fishing, bird-watching or other activities. The boats have a bow door which lowers to form a boarding ramp and the open level deck provides access throughout. A list of locations is given on its website. Contact the Director, Andy Beadsley at the above address.

Get Caravanning is an introductory guide to caravans and motor caravans for leisure use published by RADAR with the support of The Caravan Club. Available from RADAR ☎ 020 7250 3222 or on Ⓦ www.radar.org.uk

MENTAL HEALTH AND WELL-BEING

Looking after our mental – as well as physical – health is important for everyone. Things that are positive for mental well-being include having control in your own life, supportive friendships and relationships, employment or other activity where you are contributing and physical well-being (particularly exercise and being free of drug and alcohol problems).

Very many of us experience mental health problems – about one in four of the population. And millions each year get through it. Life may change as a result at first, but it is possible to 'recover' – to get your life back. At first the shock of the mental health crisis or difficulty may leave you with feelings of loss and confusion, but you can find your own path to the life you want, a life that is meaningful and fulfilling.

For some of us, the problems may be temporary. For others of us, they continue or recur. In either case a good life is not just possible, it has been achieved by many people.

Developing a mental health problem can be scary. You may have frightening thoughts or feel unable to do things you can normally do. You can seek information and advice from national Helplines and publications provided by charities like Mind or Rethink.

Because there is a lot of prejudice it can be difficult to ask for help – you may feel that makes you a failure. But that is not true. As the Rethink website puts it, 'No one is expected to be able to overcome mental health problems without support. Asking for help is not a sign of weakness. On the contrary, it takes courage…'.

Many people find it helpful to seek the support of people who have experienced similar problems or challenges - through voluntary sector organisations (e.g. Depression Alliance, MDF the bi-polar organisation) or the Expert Patient Programme.

You can seek professional help by going through a GP. A GP will often offer treatment or support directly – for instance, medication, counselling or talking therapy such as cognitive behavioural therapy - or may refer you to someone who can help with your problem. You might be referred to see a psychiatrist, or to a community mental health team (which includes people from different professions, like social work, nursing, psychology, occupational therapy, psychiatry) or to an early intervention team (for people with early experiences of mental health problems). You may be given a diagnosis: some diagnoses include depression, bi-polar disorder (or manic depression), schizophrenia, anxiety, obsessive compulsive disorder or personality difficulties. A stay in hospital may be suggested if you are very unwell.

There are many different types of medication – for instance, anti-depressants, anti-psychotic drugs, mood stabilisers.

Having information can help a lot when it comes to understanding what professionals are offering and deciding what you plan to do. Remember - except in rare circumstances (see below) it is your decision which treatments and supports you choose. It's your life: you choose.

Advocacy can also be helpful – someone to support you in advocating for what you want. It might be a friend, a family member or advocacy service.

In rare circumstances if there are risks of harm to you or others, or a serious risk to your health, it is possible for you to be placed in a hospital and/or treated against your will. If this happens you have a right to appeal to a Mental Health Review Tribunal. Mind and Rethink have information on your rights and can put you in touch with legal advisors.

One of the things that makes most difference when you experience mental health problems is keeping up your normal activities and relationships where you can – or taking some time out while you are really unwell, but leaving the door open to return. Keeping your job or college place will support your recovery – the longer you are out, the harder it can be to get back. Similarly with important relationships and friendships – you may not want to see people for a while, but keeping some contact so you can resume contact later can make a difference.

It can be good to start your activities gradually at first, with some support if you need it - but you don't need to be fully well to start working or seeing friends.

Some people are prejudiced when it comes to others experiencing mental health problems and may discriminate, for instance by not offering a job to someone because they have had psychiatric treatment. This is against the law (the Disability Discrimination Act 1995) – and discrimination is being actively challenged. A group of mental health charities have launched Time to Change, a major campaign to tackle discrimination on mental health grounds. If you have mental health problems that impact on your day to day activities over time, you have rights under the Disability Discrimination Act ('disability' is the overarching term used to cover all mental and physical health conditions and disabilities). Under this law you should not be treated 'unfavourably' - i.e. discriminated against just because you have a mental health condition; and if you require a 'reasonable adjustment' in order to work, go to school/college or use any type of services (from shops to travel) you should be able to get 'adjustments' as long as they are reasonable for the business offering them. For instance, you might need to start working again gradually (part-time at first), and at work you might need to work a different shift pattern, to have time off for medical appointments or to have contact with a mental health support worker by 'phone from work when needed. If you do face discrimination, contact the Equality and Human Rights Commission for advice.

If you have longer term mental health problems you may qualify for a number of schemes and initiatives that are for all 'disabled people'. There are schemes to help people get back into work (Access to Work, Pathways to Work. Job Centre Plus can let you know the details). There are programmes to enable disabled people to have choice and control over their own services – like individual budgets and direct payments, which mean you can manage your own care and support if you choose. You may also be entitled to disability benefits: for example, Disability Living Allowance (to help with extra costs of disability), Employment and Support Allowance (for people who face challenges in getting into work).

By arming yourself with information you can find the best route to your own, unique recovery.

The Expert Patients Programme

The Expert Patients Programme, established by the Department of Health, is a self-management programme that has been specifically developed for people living with long-term conditions. The aim of the programme is to support people in increasing their confidence, improving their quality of life and better managing their condition. The Expert Patients Programme is delivered locally by a network of trainers and around 1400 volunteer tutors with long-term conditions.

The programme focuses on five core self-management skills:
❱ problem solving
❱ decision making
❱ resource utilisation
❱ developing effective partnerships with healthcare providers

❱ and taking action

The programme offers a tool-kit of fundamental techniques that patients can undertake to improve their quality of life, living with a long-term condition.

The course enables patients to develop their communication skills, manage their emotions, manage daily activities, interact with the healthcare system, find health resources, plan for the future, understand exercising and healthy eating, and manage fatigue, sleep, pain, anger and depression.

The Expert Patients Programme Community Interest Company (EPP CIC) was created to develop, market and deliver self-management courses. For more information on the EPP CIC, to find a local course and to ask about its publications contact: EPP CIC, 32-36 Loman Street, London SE1 0EH. ☎ 020 7922 7860. @ get.info@eppcic.co.uk

Ⓦ www.expertpatients.co.uk

Useful Contacts

Depression Alliance
212 Spitfire Studios, 63 - 71 Collier Street, London N1 9BE.

☎ 0845 123 2320.
@ information@depressionalliance.org
Ⓦ www.depressionalliance.org

DA is the leading UK charity to relieve and prevent depression. It provides help and information through publications, supporter services and a network of self-help groups for people affected by depression.

Equality and Human Rights Commission
For contact details see Discrimination section

Jobcentre Plus
Jobcentre Plus offers a range of services to disabled people, people with health conditions and carers. A key feature of most of these services is the network of Disability Employment Advisers (DEAs) who provide advice on finding and keeping a job. DEAs can also provide the entry to Access to Work funds, enabling your employer to make reasonable adjustments at a relatively low cost or indeed no cost at all. The contact details can be obtained from local Jobcentre Plus offices and are listed on www.jobcentreplus.com

MDF – The BiPolar Organisation
Castle Works, 21 St. George's Road, London SE1 6ES.

☎ 08456 340540
Ⓦ www.mdf.org.uk

MDF works to enable people affected by bipolar disorder (manic depression) to take control of their lives. The range of services offered includes a wide range of publications, support and development of self-help opportunities and an eCommunity to communicate with others on bipolar related topics.

Mind
15-19 Broadway, London E15 4BQ.

☎ 0845 766 0163 (MindInfoLine)
or 020 8519 2122.

@ contact@mind.org.uk
Ⓦ www.mind.org.ukMind Cymru

3rd Floor, Quebec House, Castlebridge, 5-19 Cowbridge Road East, Cardiff CF11 9AB.

☎ 029 2039 5123.

Mind is the leading mental health charity in England and Wales. It offers a telephone information line, publications and support networks for users of mental health services. Local Mind associations (LMAs) provide a range of services.

In Scotland, a similar organisation is:

Scottish Association for Mental Health, Cumbrae House,
15 Carlton Court, Glasgow G5 9JP.
☎ 0141 568 7000.
@ enquire@samh.org.uk
Ⓦ www.samh.org.uk

Rethink
89 Albert Embankment, London SE1 7TP.
☎ 0845 456 0455.
@ info@rethink.org
Ⓦ www.rethink.org

Rethink works to help everyone affected by severe mental illness recover a better quality of life. It provides support with information, advice, services, groups, campaigns and research. Expert advice on issues affecting the lives of people living with mental illness is available from its National Advisory Service on 020 7840 3188 or advice@rethink.org

SANE
1st Floor, Cityside House, 40 Adler Street, London E1 1EE.
☎ 020 7375 1002.
@ info@sane.org.uk
Ⓦ www.sane.org.uk

SANE raises awareness of mental illness, campaigns to improve services, and initiates and funds research into the causes of serious mental illness. It also provides information and support to those experiencing mental health problems through its SANEline helpline, available 6pm-11pm every day on 0845 767 8000 or its SANEmail at sanemail@sane.org.uk

Stand to Reason
@ info@standtoreason.org.uk
Ⓦ www.standtoreason.org.uk

Stand to Reason is a service-user led organisation that intends to work with and for people with mental ill health. It aims to raise the profile, fight prejudice, establish rights and achieve equality for people who have experience of mental distress and ill health.

Time To Change
15-19 Broadway, London E15 4BQ.
☎ 020 8215 2356.
@ info@time-to-change.org.uk
Ⓦ www.time-to-change.org.uk

Time to Change is a partnership of organisations to end mental health discrimination. The programme, consisting of 35 projects, is run by Mental Health Media, Mind and Rethink and evaluated by the Institute of Psychiatry at King's College.

The UK Advocacy Network (UKAN)
Volserve House, 14 - 18 West Bar Green, Sheffield S1 2DA.
@ office@u-kan.co.uk
Ⓦ www.u-kan.co.uk

UKAN is a user controlled national federation of advocacy projects, patients' councils, user forums and self-help and support groups working in the field of mental health. UKAN offers information, training and support on the improvement of mental health services.

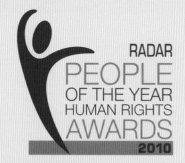

RADAR
PEOPLE
OF THE YEAR
HUMAN RIGHTS
AWARDS
2010

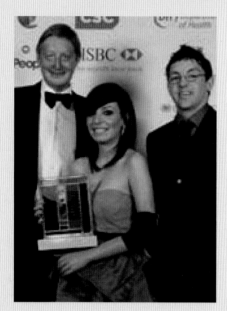

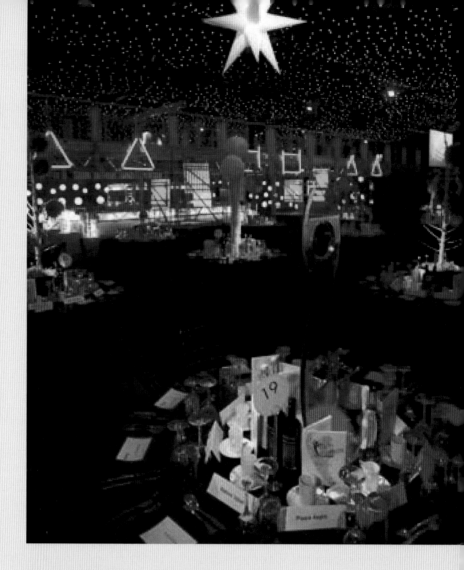

"People of the Year Awards is a highlight in the calendar for high level people and businesses on the disability agenda – it's excellent exposure for us"

Citigroup

RADAR – Unique in recognising remarkable people

Now in it's 44th year and the only event of it's kind in Europe, RADAR's inspiring People of the Year Awards, honours people who have made giant inroads into disability equality.

Last year's event was hosted by Frank Gardner OBE with a 'Future Proofing Disability Equality' Theme and 620 people attended. Read about last year's winners at www.radar.org.uk and find out how you can sponsor or support this event by e-mailing **radar@radar.org.uk**

MOTORING

For most people it's vital to be independently mobile and for many disabled people this need is met by a vehicle which is often adapted to their particular needs, whether as a driver or passenger.

Driving Licences

Disabled people, with the higher rate mobility component of DLA can obtain a provisional driving licence from the age of 16.

All applicants for a licence must declare to the Driver & Vehicle Licensing Agency (DVLA) any existing disability or medical condition affecting their fitness to drive. Existing licence holders are legally required to inform DVLA if they have acquired a disability or if there is a deterioration or change in any existing disability or medical condition. If a disability is stable and non-progressive, a licence will normally be valid until the age of 70; otherwise a licence may be restricted to one, two or three years. It is possible to apply to renew a restricted licence when it expires.

There are some medical conditions that will usually mean that someone is judged unfit to drive. These are:

- epilepsy, unless the applicant has been free of seizures for a year, or for the previous three years has only had seizures when asleep;

- severe mental disorder;

- liability to sudden attacks of giddiness or fainting;

- inability to read a normal number plate at a distance of 20.5m in good daylight, with the aid of spectacles or contact lenses if usually worn;

- persistent drug or alcohol misuse;

- any other disability likely to cause the driver to be a danger to the public.

For further information contact the DVLA,
Drivers Medical Group,
Swansea SA99 1DL.
☎ 0870 600 0301. Textphone: 01792 766366.   @ eftd@dvla.gsi.gov.uk
Ⓦ www.dvla.gov.uk

In Northern Ireland –
DVLNI, Driver Licensing Division,
County Hall, Castlerock Road, Coleraine BT51 3TB. ☎ 0845 402 4000.
Textphone: 028 7034 1380. Ⓦ www.dvlni.gov.uk

Driving Lessons

All new drivers are strongly advised to have professional driving lessons at least at the beginning of their learning period. There are many driving instructors with experience and training in this field, who as well as teaching driving skills know about techniques for transferring between a car and a wheelchair, operating, adapted controls, etc. Disability motoring organisations and mobility centres (see later in this section) can provide information on appropriately trained instructors.

It is possible to have lessons in a privately owned, adapted car. However some driving schools and instructors have cars fitted with at least simple hand controls.

For people intending to get a car through Motability, grants towards the cost of driving lessons may be available.

The BSM Mobility Service has around 200 instructors who have received mobility training as well as being licensed by the Driving Standards Agency. Automatic cars with dual controls and some common adaptations are used and additional equipment can be provided if required. For further information ☎ 0845 727 6276. Ⓦ www.bsm.co.uk/mobility

Driving Tests

The driving test is in two parts: theory and practical. The theory tests are taken in test centres. These are usually accessible, but if there are any access problems arrangements can be made to have the test at another centre or elsewhere. Arrangements can also be made to assist people who would have difficulty operating the computer screen. The test is carried out in 21 languages and BSL can be shown on the screen. Advance notice needs to be given for this when applying for the test.

Disabled people are given priority when booking the practical test. Additional time is allotted so that the examiner can be informed of the nature and function of any adaptations, to allow for extra time to get in and out of the car or any other reasons. Deaf people can take an interpreter with them, who must be over 16 and not a driving instructor. The Driving Standards Agency asks anyone who has any disability that may affect their driving or their taking of the test to let them know when booking the practical test. Information is available on
ꟽ www.dsa.gov.uk

Driving Assessments and Vehicle Adaptations

A wide range of accessories and forms of adaptations are available which can affect the way in which disabled people can use their cars. As new equipment is constantly being introduced it can be useful for even experienced disabled drivers to check on what is available from time to time, perhaps when replacing an existing car. For a new driver or one whose abilities have changed an assessment is strongly recommended.

Ricability, with funding from the Department of Transport, has published independent guides on Choosing a Car, Car Controls, People Lifters and Getting a Wheelchair into a Car and Getting In and Out of a Car. It also has seven guides on car choice and adaptations for people with specific impairments or conditions. Contact Ricability, 30 Angel Gate, City Road, London EC1V 2PT.
☎ 020 7427 2460.
Textphone: 020 7427 2469. ꟽ www.ricability.org.uk

Mobility Centres

Advice on motoring for disabled and elderly people can be obtained from Mobility Centres located around the country. All provide an information service with advice on cars, adaptations and special equipment for drivers and for passengers. Some offer other services such as driving instruction or carrying out adaptations. The following are members of the Forum of Mobility Centres ☎ 0800 559 3636, ꟽ www.mobility-centres.org.uk:

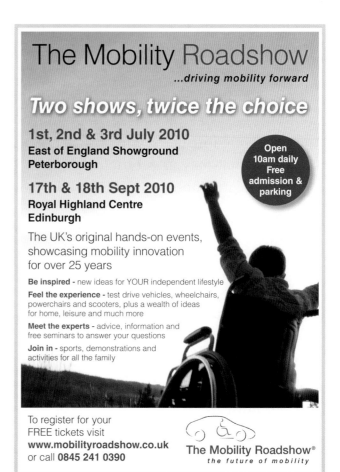
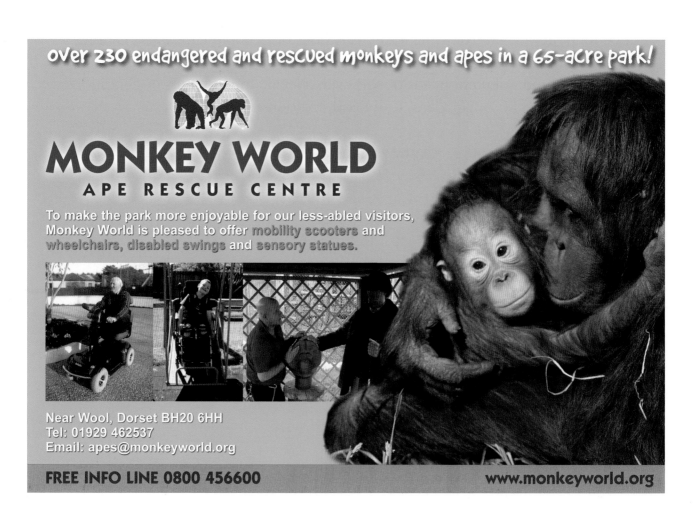

Belfast – Northern Ireland Mobility Centre

Disability Action, Portside Business Park, 189 Airport Road, Belfast BT3 9ED.
☎ 028 9029 7880.
Textphone: 029 9029 7882.
@ mobilitycentre@disabilityaction.org

Birmingham - Regional Driving Assessment Centre

Unit 11 Network Park, Duddeston Mill Road, Birmingham B8 1AU.
☎ 0845 337 1540.
@ info@rdac.co.uk
Ⓦ www.rdac.co.uk

Bristol - Mobility Service of the Disabled Living Centre (West of England)

The Vassall Centre, Gill Avenue, Fishponds, Bristol BS16 2QQ.
☎ 0117 965 9353.
@ mobserv@yhisisliving.org.uk
Ⓦ www.thisisliving.org.uk

Cardiff - South Wales Mobility & Driving Assessment Service

Rookwood Hospital, Fairwater Road, Llandaff, Cardiff CF5 2YN.
☎ 029 2055 5130.
@ helen@wddac.co.uk

Carshalton - Queen Elizabeth's Foundation Mobility Centre

Damson Drive, Fountain Drive, Carshalton, Surrey SM5 4NR.
☎ 020 8770 1151.
@ info@mobility-qe.org
Ⓦ www.qefd.org/mobilitycentre

Denbighshire - North Wales Mobility & Driving Assessment Service

Glan Clwyd Hospital, Bodelwyddan, Denbighshire LL18 5UJ.
☎ 01745 584858.
@ alexbarr@btconnect.com

Derby – DrivAbility

Kingsway Hospital, Kingsway, Derby DE22 3LZ.
☎ 01332 371829.
@ driving@derbyhospitals.nhs.uk
Ⓦ www.derbydrivability.com

Edinburgh - Scottish Driving Assessment Service

Astley Ainslie Hospital, 133 Grange Loan, Edinburgh EH9 2HL.
☎ 0131 537 9192.
@ marlene.mackenzie@lpct.scot.nhs.uk

Leeds - William Merritt Disabled Living Centre & Mobility Service

St Mary's Hospital, Green Hill Road, Armley, Leeds LS12 3QE.
☎ 0113 305 5288.
@ mobility.service@nhs.net
Ⓦ www.williammerrittleeds.org

Maidstone - DART Driving Assessment & Advice Centre

Cobtree Ward, Preston Hall Hospital, London Road, Aylesford, Kent ME20 7NJ.
☎ 01622 795719.
@ julie.chatburn@nhs.net

Newcastle upon Tyne – North East Drive Mobility

Walkergate Park, Centre for Neuro-rehabilitation & Neuro-psychiatry, Benfield Road,
Newcastle upon Tyne NE6 4QD.
☎ 0191 287 5090.
@ northeast.drivemobility@ntw.nhs.uk

Oxford – Oxford Mobility Centre

(contact via the Birmingham Centre above)

Southampton – Southampton Mobility Centre

Unit 211 Solent Business Centre, Millbrook Road West, Southampton SO15 0HW.
☎ 023 8051 2222.
@ admin@sotoncentre.co.uk

Thetford - Kilverstone Mobility Assessment Centre

2 Napier Place, Thetford, Norfolk IP24 3RL.
☎ 01842 753029.
@ mail@kmacmobil.org.uk
Ⓦ www.kmacmobil.org.uk

Truro - Cornwall Mobility Centre

Tehidy House, Royal Cornwall Hospital, Truro TR1 3LJ.
☎ 01872 254920.
@ mobility@rcht.cornwall.nhs.uk
Ⓦ www.cornwallmobilitycentre.co.uk

Welwyn Garden City - Hertfordshire Action on Disability Mobility Centre

The Woodside Centre, The Commons, Welwyn Garden City AL7 4DD.
☎ 01707 324581.
@ driving@hadnet.co.uk
Ⓦ www.hadnet.org.uk

Wigan - Wrightington Mobility Centre

Wrightington Hospital, Hall Lane, Appley Bridge, Wigan WN6 9EP.
☎ 01257 256409.
@ mobility.centre@alwpct.nhs.uk

A wide range of equipment, large and small, is available to make a car easier for a disabled person to use. As examples:

Autoadapt UK Ltd

Unit 4 Windsor Industrial Estate, Rupert Street, Aston, Birmingham B7 4PR.
☎ 0121 333 5170.
Ⓦ www.autoadapt.co.uk

Offers a range of products which assist in getting in and out of a car through a network of dealers. Its latest product is a seat that swivels and tilts to maximise the headroom and has a footrest to avoid the need to lift the legs over the door opening.

CG-Lock

Suite 202, 1 Deansgate, Manchester M3 1AZ.
☎ 0161 832 3786. Ⓦ www.cg-lock.co.uk

Originally developed for high performance driving, the CG-Lock clips on a standard seat belt and provides greater stability by securing the driver's hips against the seat. It requires no structural alteration to the car or existing seatbelt and can be fitted in a few minutes. The CG-Lock can be tested at Mobility Centres.

National Mobility Equipment Dealers Association

☎ 01784 470860. Ⓦ www.nmedauk.org

NMEDA (UK) is a trade association representing companies that adapt cars and provide specialist equipment.

Mobility Roadshow

The annual Mobility Roadshow provides the opportunity to view and test drive a wide range of adapted cars and other vehicles, see mobility products and talk to voluntary organisations. This takes place in June every year at a venue in central England and every other year near Edinburgh in April. For information on dates and venues contact Mobility Choice, MacAdam Avenue, Crowthorne Business Estate, Old Wokingham Road, Crowthorne, Berks RG45 6XD.
☎ 0845 241 0390.
Ⓦ www.mobilityroadshow.co.uk

Motability
Warwick House, Roydon Road, HarlowEssex CM19 5PX
☎ 0800 093 1000. Textphone: 01279 632213. ⓦ www.motability.co.uk
People receiving the higher rate mobility component of the Disability Living
Allowance or the War Pensioners Mobility Supplement can use Motability to
acquire a car. This can be by contract hire leasing of a new car over a 3-year
period or hire purchase of a new or used car over 2 or 5 years. Motability works
with around 4000 approved dealers around the UK. Under a related scheme,
powered buggies and wheelchairs can be leased or bought on hire purchase.

Tax, Insurance & Other Matters

People who receive the higher rate mobility component of Disability Living
Allowance are eligible to apply for exemption from Vehicle Excise Duty (road tax).
Exemption forms must be obtained from the Disability & Carer Benefits Directorate
and sent to the DVLA with the car logbook. Detailed information can be obtained
from a local DVLA Vehicle Registration Office or on ⓦ www.dvla.gov.uk

Some specialist vehicles and adaptations to vehicles can be zero rated for VAT
when provided for disabled people. The supplier should have details of these for
which information is given in Vat Notice 701/59 from HM Revenue and Customs.

Insurers cannot charge higher premiums for disabled motorists unless the extra
charge is based on factual, statistical data or there are other relevant factors to
indicate that there is a higher risk. A number of brokers and insurance companies
specialise in motor insurance for disabled drivers and information on these can be
obtained from disability motoring organisations.

Although there often are concessions for disabled motorists in respect of road,
tunnel and bridge tolls and other charges such as the Congestion Charge in
central London, and ferry fares these follow no standard pattern. Information
can be obtained from the individual operators or from the disability motoring
organisations.

'Get Motoring' is a free RADAR booklet giving practical guidance for disabled motorists on finding and financing a car. Available from RADAR ☎ 020 7250 3222. Textphone: 020 7250 4119. Ⓦ www.radar.org.uk

Parking

The Blue Badge Scheme provides a national system of on-street parking concessions for people with severe mobility problems. Badge holders can park without charge at parking meters and in pay-and-display bays, are exempt from time limits imposed on others and may park for up to 3 hours on yellow lines, except where loading or other restrictions apply.

The scheme is administered by local authorities in England, Scotland and Wales and the Roads Service in Northern Ireland. It is available to those who:

❯ receive the Mobility Component of the Disability Living Allowance or the War Pensioners Mobility Supplement;

❯ are a registered blind person;

❯ have a severe disability in both upper limbs, regularly drive a car and are unable to use a parking meter or have great difficulty in doing so;

❯ are aged under 2 and need to travel with bulky medical equipment or be close to a vehicle for medical treatment; or

❯ have a permanent and substantial disability which causes the inability to walk or very considerable difficulty in walking.

The scheme does not apply in parts of the centre of London where 4 local authorities have their own schemes, although there are some parking spaces provided for Blue Badge holders visiting the area.

Although the Blue Badge Scheme does not apply to off-street parking, it is often used by local authorities as the basis for concessionary use of car parks and to indicate that designated parking bays in privately owned parking areas are being used correctly.

An interactive map is now available showing parking bays for Blue Badge holders in 100 major towns and cities across the UK including London. It also indicates parking bays on red routes in London and accessible petrol stations and much other information. Any time restrictions or other special features of the parking bays are shown on the map, which is available on **www.direct.gov.uk/ bluebadgemap**

The Blue Badge can be used, with care, in some other countries. Official reciprocal arrangements have been made with 29 European countries. This means that a British badge holder can make use of the national parking concessions available to disabled people in the other country. A leaflet outlining these can be down loaded from www.iam.org.uk. In other countries, in which there may not be any national scheme, the use of the Blue Badge will often be acceptable.

Blue Badge Network
198 Wolverhampton Street,
Dudley DY1 1DZ.
☎ 01384 257001.
@ headoffice@bluebadgenetwork.org.uk
Ⓦ www.bluebadgenetwork.org.uk

The Blue Badge Network is a membership organisation aiming to help disabled people and, in particular, to maintain the integrity of the concessionary parking permit.

Disability Motoring Organisations

Mobilise
National Headquarters, Ashwellthorpe, Norwich NR16 1EX.
☎ 01508 489449.
@ enquiries@mobilise.info
Ⓦ www.mobilise.info

Mobilise campaigns and provides information on all matters related to motoring/ mobility and disabled people.

Disabled Motorists' Federation

c/o 145 Knoulberry Road, Blackfell,
Washington NE37 1JN.
☎ 0191 416 3172.
Ⓦ www.dmfnet.co.uk

National Association for Bikers with a Disability

Unit 20, The Bridgewater Centre,
Robson Avenue, Urmston, Manchester
M41 7TE. ☎ 0844 415 4849.
@ nabd@nabd.org.uk
Ⓦ www.nabd.org.uk

NABD caters for disabled people
who want to enjoy the freedom of
motorcycling. It provides a range of
services for its members including
advice and help on training, licensing,
adaptations, insurance and the costs
of adaptations. It has a network of
local representatives and produces a
quarterly magazine.

General Motoring Organisations

AA (Automobile Association)
Contact Centre, Lambert House,
Stockport Road, Cheadle SK8 2DY.
☎ 0800 262050 (Disability Helpline),
0870 550 0600.
Textphone: 0800 328 2810.
Ⓦ theaa.com

Green Flag Motoring Assistance

Cote Lane, Leeds LS28 5GF.
☎ 0800 000111 (Helpline),
0113 390 4000.
Textphone: 0800 800 610
Ⓦ www.greenflag.co.uk

Green Flag customers who cannot use
a telephone because of impaired hearing
or speech can use a dedicated text
messaging number when they need to
use the breakdown service.

RAC Motoring Services

Great Park Road, Bradley Stoke, Bristol
BS32 4QN.
☎ 0870 572 2722.
Ⓦ www.rac.co.uk

PUBLIC TOILETS

Traditionally, public conveniences have been provided by local authorities. In many areas there was a long history of the inclusion within them of features for disabled people, although the actual design or fittings varied in effectiveness. However, there are still examples of inaccessible public conveniences still being in use.

Over recent years there have been significant changes in the ways in which toilets in public places are provided and managed affecting the ways that people can either find out what is available or suggest improvements. In many instances the cleaning and routine maintenance will have been contracted out. In some cases the responsibility for certain types of toilets, for example those in parks, markets and those on the streets have been split between different departments. Pre-built, self-cleaning toilets (sometimes referred to as "automatic" or "superloos") have been installed in an increasing number of locations where they are maintained by the supplier. In some districts the responsibility for public conveniences has been handed over to other bodies such as Parish Councils or to private companies managing elements of town centres. Community Toilet schemes have been established in some areas where the local authority has arranged for the public to be able to use toilets in some privately owned places such as pubs and cafes. Finally the toilets inside the growing number of shopping centres and other semi-public areas are usually the responsibility of the owners or managers of the premises.

Overall there has been a reduction in the number of traditional public conveniences operated by local authorities, although this is only recently affected unisex units designed for disabled people, as councils have cut expenditure. However, recently as a result of greater awareness and the impact of Building Regulations and the Disability Discrimination Act, appropriately designed toilets have become more common in privately owned buildings used by the public such as large shops, restaurants and bars and also in public premises including parks and libraries. Where these are provided for customers many people may choose to patronise those places where they can use the toilet if necessary.

The "Just Can't Wait" Card is for people who may need to get to a toilet quickly when a public one is not available. The idea is that it would be shown in a shop or other establishment as a request to use a staff or other toilet. There is no guarantee that the request would be granted, although some high street names have signed up to accept it, or that the toilet available would have any particular features. The Card and other information are available from Bladder & Bowel Foundation, ☎ 0870 770 3246. @ info@bladderandbowelfoundation.org

National Key Scheme for Toilets for Disabled People

The National Key Scheme, sometimes referred to as the RADAR key scheme, is widely used throughout the UK on toilets designed for disabled people. It was introduced 25 years ago because an increasing number of local authorities and other bodies were locking their toilets for disabled people to counter vandalism and misuse, or delaying the provision of new toilets until some security system was available.

If toilets have to be locked, providers are asked to fit the standard NKS lock and to make keys available to disabled people in their area. Whenever possible a key should be held nearby for disabled people who have not got one with them. The scheme has now been adopted by over 400 local authorities and the NKS lock has also been fitted to toilets provided by a wide range of other organisations including transport undertakings, pub companies, visitor attractions, shops and community organisations.

When the scheme was introduced RADAR agreed to maintain a list of the toilets fitted with the NKS lock. This is up-dated regularly and published as the "National Key Scheme Guide", available price £12.25 including postage & packing.

If disabled people cannot obtain a key locally, they can get one from RADAR by sending £3.50 and a simple statement that they need it because they are disabled or that it is to be used by a disabled person. It can also be ordered on www.radar. org.uk

Changing Places Toilets

Some disabled people need facilities beyond those found in a "standard" toilet designed for disabled people. Changing Places toilets have

❯ An adjustable height adult changing table

❯ A hoist with tracking, or mobile a mobile one if necessary

❯ Space both sides of the WC for assistants.

As yet there are very few Changing Places toilets around the country and most are only available when the premises in which they are situated are open. For further information about Changing Places, including a list of current and planned locations call ☎ 020 7696 6019 or in Scotland ☎ 01382 385154 or see Ⓦ www.changing-places.org

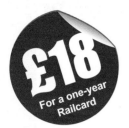

£18 For a one-year Railcard

Get 1/3 off rail fares for you...

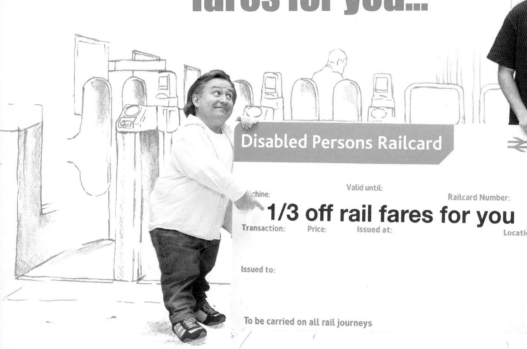

Disabled Persons Railcard

Valid until:

Railcard Number:

1/3 off rail fares for you

Transaction: Price: Issued at: Location:

Issued to:

To be carried on all rail journeys

...and a companion...

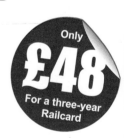

Only **£48** For a three-year Railcard

You qualify if you meet any one of the criteria below:

✓ You receive Attendance Allowance

✓ You receive Disability Living Allowance (at either the higher or lower rate for getting around or the higher or middle rate for personal care)

✓ You are registered as having a visual impairment

✓ You have epilepsy and have repeated attacks or are currently prohibited from driving because of epilepsy

✓ You are registered as deaf or use a hearing aid

✓ You receive severe disablement allowance

✓ You receive War Pensioner's Mobility Supplement for 80% or more disability

✓ You are buying or leasing a vehicle through the Motability scheme

To find out how to apply see the leaflet 'Rail Travel Made Easy' (available at stations) or contact us:

 Web
www.disabledpersons-railcard.co.uk

 Email
disability@atoc.org

 Telephone
0845 605 0525

 Textphone
0845 601 0132

PUBLIC TRANSPORT

In the past public transport systems were developed with little or no regard to the needs of disabled people. This is now changing particularly as transport regulations under the Disability Discrimination Act come into effect. However, progress is patchy both geographically and between various forms of transport.

Travel Planning

Advance planning is often needed and, if assistance may be required at any point in the journey, advance notification will usually be required. Over most of England and Wales, county and unitary councils have public transport responsibilities and have a Public Transport Information Officer. Some publish specific information for disabled passengers.

In the major conurbations this oversight is carried out by Passenger Transport Executives and in London by Transport for London.

GMPTE
9 Portland Street, Piccadilly Gardens, Manchester M60 1HX.
☎ 0871 200 2233.
Textphone: 0870 241 2216.
Ⓦ www.gmpte.com

MerseyTravel
24 Hatton Garden, Liverpool L3 2AN.
☎/Textphone 0151 227 5181.
Ⓦ www.merseytravel.gov.uk

Metro
Wellington House, 40-50 Wellington Street, Leeds LS1 2DE.
☎ 0113 251 7272.
Ⓦ www.wymetro.com

Network West Midlands
Centro House, 16 Summer Lane, Birmingham B19 3SD.
☎ 0121 200 2700.
Textphone: 0121 214 7777.
Ⓦ www.networkwestmidlands.com

Nexus
Nexus House, St James Boulevard, Newcastle upon Tyne NE1 4AX.
☎ 0191 2020 500.
Textphone: 0191 2020 501.
Ⓦ www.nexus.org.uk

South Yorkshire PTE
11 Broad Street, Sheffield S1 2BQ.
☎ 0114 276 7575.
Ⓦ www.sypte.co.uk

Transport for London
Travel Information, 55 Broadway,
London SW1H OBD.
☎ 020 7222 1234.
Textphone: 020 7918 3015.
@ travinfo@tfl.gov.uk
Ⓦ www.tfl.gov.uk

In Northern Ireland rail and bus services are overseen by:

Translink, Central Station
Belfast BT1 3PB.
☎ 028 9066 6630.
Textphone: 028 9035 4007.
Ⓦ www.translink.co.uk

In Scotland, transport planning is carried out by Regional Transport Partnerships, some of whom also have more direct transport functions. RTPs are:

Shetland TP
11 Hill Lane, Lerwick ZE1 OHA.
☎ 01595 744868.
Ⓦ www.shetland.gov.uk/transport

Highlands & Islands RTP
Building 25, Inverness Airport,
Inverness IV2 7JB.
☎ 01667 460464
Ⓦ www.hitrans.org.uk

North East RTP
27-29 King Street, Aberdeen AB24 5AN.
☎ 01224 625524.
Ⓦ www.nestrans.org.uk

Tayside & Central RTP
Bordeaux House, 31 Kinnoull Street,
Perth PH1 5EN.
☎ 01738 475775.
Ⓦ www.tactran.gov.uk

South East RTP
1st Floor, 8B MacDonald Road,
Edinburgh EH7 4LZ.
☎ 0131 524 5150.
Ⓦ www.sestran.gov.uk

Strathclyde PT
Consort House, 12 West George Street,
Glasgow G2 1HA.
☎ 0141 332 6811
Ⓦ www.spt.co.uk

South West PT
c/o Dumfries & Galloway Council,
Kirkbank House, English Street,
Dumfries DG1 2HS.
☎ 01387 260102.
Ⓦ www.dumgal.gov.uk/rtpb

Nationally, general information on transport services and timetables is available through Traveline ☎ 0870 608 2608.
Textphone: 0870 241 2216.
Ⓦ www.traveline.org.uk

www.transportdirect.info is a transport planning website that includes options for using all types of public transport and private motoring for point-to-point journeys in Great Britain.

www.dptac.gov.uk/door-to-door is a regularly up-dated source of information for disabled people on all forms of transport.

Ricability has published Wheels Within Wheels, a guide to using a wheelchair on public transport. Information is available from Ricability, 30 Angel Gate, City Road, London EC1V 2PT.
☎ 020 7427 2460.
Textphone: 020 7427 2469.
Ⓦ www.ricability.org.uk

Air Travel

With air travel being an international industry some attitudes and practises that are outdated in the UK can still be encountered in the airlines of some other countries. Other factors that can make air travel more complicated for disabled passengers and lead to their need for assistance can arise from security requirements, design and safety features of aircraft, the size of airports and, for many people, unfamiliarity with the environment.

Under EC Regulation 1107/206 it is illegal for an airline, travel agent or tour operator to refuse a booking on the grounds of disability or to refuse to embark a disabled person who has a valid ticket and reservation. In Britain anyone who has been refused boarding on the grounds of disability or reduced mobility will be able to complain initially to the Equalities & Human Rights Commission (EHRC). The Commission will advise them on their rights and could refer the matter to the Civil Aviation Authority (CAA) which will have power to prosecute. An airline found guilty could face an unlimited fine. Airport managing bodies are also required to organise the provision of the services necessary to enable disabled/reduced mobility passengers to board, disembark and transit between flights.

Airlines generally have established procedures for assisting disabled passengers. Most people, particularly those with permanent and stable conditions, will not require medical clearance before travelling. However, this may vary between airlines and clearance will generally be required for certain conditions, including some that may have little effect in other situations. It is important to check at the time of booking what, if any, medical information will be required.

Most airports are physically accessible and many have introduced facilities and services to make it easier for disabled people to use them. However, most airport terminals are large, complex premises so finding facilities and assistance may be difficult. Often airports have information for disabled people on their website and some have a separately published access guide.

Wheelchair users should be able to stay in their own wheelchairs until boarding, and other people given such assistance as they need to reach the departure gate. Depending on the airline and the size of the aircraft there may be an on-board wheelchair for transfer to the seat. It may be possible to request a seat in a particular area, say near a toilet or with more leg room. However, the seats beside emergency exits, which do have more space, will be allocated to people who are perceived as having the dexterity and strength to open the doors if necessary.

Most pieces of equipment required by a disabled passenger are carried free of charge. Larger items, including wheelchairs, are carried in the hold although smaller items can be taken into the cabin. Information should be sought from the airline on any equipment, particularly if it may be required during the flight.

As with other forms of transport, if any assistance or service may be necessary it should be requested in advance. A complication with air travel is that more organisations may be involved than with other forms of transport, particularly if the flight is by a charter aircraft as part of a holiday package. In most cases requested arrangements are carried out but when things do go wrong it is often the result of a failure in the communication chain. It is therefore advisable to check that appropriate messages have been passed on and emphasise the importance of the requests.

More detailed information is included in 'Access to Air Travel: Guidance for disabled and less mobile passengers', which was issued by the Disabled Persons Transport Advisory Committee in 2003. It is available from DPTAC Secretariat, Great Minster House, 76 Marsham Street, London SW1P 4DR. ☎ 020 7944 8011. Textphone: 020 7944 3277. Ⓦ www.dptac.gov.uk

---

Bus & Coach Travel

For many years bus travel was among the least accessible form of public transport for disabled people. However things are changing. Regulations now require all new buses to be equipped with lifts or ramps with a level floor to a space to carry a passenger in a wheelchair and incorporate features such as colour contrasted handrails, easy to operate bell-pushes, etc. However, older vehicles will continue to be in use for years.

Information on routes normally served by accessible buses should be available from a Public Transport Information Office, a PTE or from the individual bus company. Although all the boarding features of a modern bus may work well at bus stations or other dedicated bus stands, there can be problems at roadside bus stops if the vehicle does not pull in sufficiently close to the footpath, if one exists, perhaps because of road works or badly parked cars.

There has been slower progress in making scheduled long-distance coach travel accessible to wheelchair users although since 2005 new coaches are be equipped with lifts.

Goldline, the express coach service between towns and cities in Northern Ireland, uses wheelchair accessible coaches on an increasing number of its services.

National Express is introducing a new vehicle in which a lift is incorporated at the main entrance and which has a space for a passenger in a wheelchair. On other services, for passengers who can manage the entrance steps, assistance can be given with advance notice and folded manual wheelchairs carried. Information is available from the National Express Disabled Peoples' Helpline on ☎ 0121 423 8479; Textphone: 0121 455 0086 or see www.nationalexpress.com.

Oxford Tube, which runs regular, scheduled services between Oxford and London, has introduced 25 low floor coaches each of which has one space for a passenger travelling in a wheelchair. For further information ☎ 01865 772250 or
Ⓦ www.oxfordtube.com

Scottish Citylink has wheelchair accessible coaches on its regular service between Edinburgh and Glasgow. For information call ☎ 0870b550 5050 or see www.citylink.co.uk

Rather more common are adapted coaches for private hire by groups which may also be used for package tours or sight-seeing trips. Information on firms with these should be available from a Public Transport Information Office or PTE.

Door-to-Door and Community Transport

Special transport schemes for people who are not able to use public transport exist in some localities. They go under a variety of names including "dial-a-ride" and "ring-and-ride", however the principle is that a disabled person can phone up to book an adapted vehicle to carry them on a specific door-to-door journey. The demand for such a service is always likely to exceed the resources available for it so a variety of restrictions are likely to be in place – people may be limited to a number of journeys in any given period of time, journeys may be limited to a particular administrative area, etc.

More general Community Transport schemes exist where no public transport is available, often but not exclusively in rural areas. Very often vehicles used for community transport will be accessible to disabled passengers.

Essentially all special transport schemes are locally run with their own priorities. Information should be available from a Public Transport Information Office.

Community Transport Association UK
Highbank, Halton Street, Hyde, Cheshire SK14 2NY.
☎ 0870 774 3586. ⓦ www.ctauk.org

CTA UK gives advice and support on establishing and improving community transport schemes and provides training.

British Red Cross branches offer a transport service for people who cannot get about easily or use public transport. It helps people to get to medical appointments, go shopping, or just to get out of the house. Contact details of local Red Cross Branches are in local phone books or can be obtained from British Red Cross, 44 Moorfields, London EC2Y 9AL. ☎ 0870 170 7000. ⓦ www.redcross.org.uk

Ferry Travel

Ferries can vary from large, modern ships used on international journeys, which may be accessible with lifts between decks, toilets designed for disabled people and adapted cabins, through to much simpler vessels on estuary crossings with open car decks that may be accessible by virtue of their lack of facilities and the short space of time that they are used. Between these extremes there are a variety of degrees of provision.

One factor that is important to remember on all tidal waters, including some quite a long way from the open sea, e.g. London, is that the gradient of any boarding ramp will vary according to the state of the tide and on occasion may be very steep.

If anyone needs assistance or information they should get in touch with the ferry operator in advance. Contact details and other information can be obtained from the public transport information points or motoring organisations.

Rail Travel

All new trains since 1998 have had to incorporate access features for disabled people, including spaces for passengers travelling in manual wheelchairs, appropriate toilets and signage. Many trains introduced before that date also have spaces for passengers in wheelchairs. Older rolling stock is being phased out but does still exist.

Train stations represent the whole range of levels of accessibility for disabled passengers. Although there has been an active process of adapting premises, it is lengthy and been concentrated on larger stations and those which were being modernised in any event. There still remain many smaller stations where the approach to one or more platforms is by steps.

In planning a journey by rail it's often easier to take through services across a major population centres rather than changing trains. Information on services and disruptions can be obtained from the National Train Enquiries ☎ 08457 484950. Textphone: 0845 605 0600. Ⓦ www.nationalrail.co.uk

Despite continuing improvements, the railway system still has problem areas and many disabled passengers will need help at some points of their journey. Anyone who may need assistance is asked to give as much advance notice as possible. Requests for information and assistance should be made to the Train Operating Company with whom you will be starting your journey on the following numbers:

Arriva Trains Wales
☎ 0845 300 3005;
Textphone: 0847 758 5469

C2C
☎ 01702 357640;
Textphone 0845 712 5988

Chiltern Railways
☎ 0845 600 5165;
Textphone: 0845 707 8051

Cross Country
☎ 0844 811 0125;
Textphone: 0844 811 0126

East Midlands Trains
☎ 0845 712 5678;
Textphone: 0845 707 8051

First Capital Connect
☎ 0800 058 2844;
Textphone: 0800 975 1052

First Great Western
☎ 0800 197 1329;
Textphone: 0800 294 9209

First ScotRail
☎ 0800 912 2901;
Textphone: 0800 912 2899

First TransPennine
☎ 0800 107 2149.
Textphone: 0800 107 2061

Gatwick Express
☎ /Textphone: 0845 850 1530

Grand Central Railway
☎ 0845 603 4852

Heathrow Express
☎ 0845 600 1515

Hull Trains
☎ 0845 071 0222;
Textphone: 0845 678 6867

Island Line
☎ 0800 528 2100;
Textphone: 0800 692 0792

London Midland
☎ 0870 092 4260. Textphone: 0845 707 8051

London Overground
☎ 0870 601 4867

Merseyrail
☎/Textphone 0151 702 2071

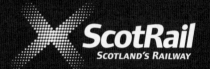
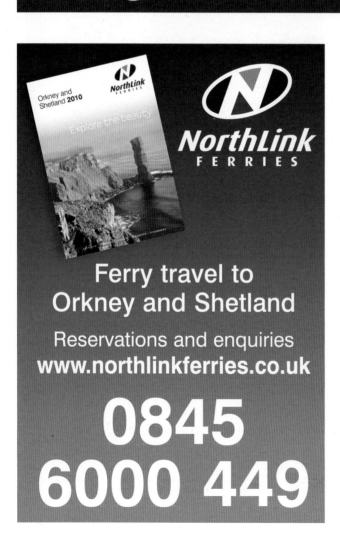
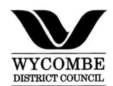

National Express East Anglia
☎ 0800 028 2878.
Textphone: 0845 606 7245

National Express East Coast
☎ 0845 722 5444;
Textphone: 0856 720 2067

Northern Rail
☎ 0845 600 8008;
Textphone: 0845 604 5608

SouthEastern
☎ 0800 783 4524;
Textphone: 0800 783 4548

South West Trains
☎ 0800 528 2100;
Textphone: 0800 692 0792

Southern
☎ 0800 138 1016;
Textphone: 0800 138 1018

Virgin Trains
☎ 0845 744 3366;
Textphone: 0845 744 3367

Wrexham & Shropshire
☎ /Textphone 0845 260 5200

The Disabled Person's Railcard gives a third off many rail fares for the cardholder and an adult travelling companion. The qualifying criteria and an application form are included in the "Rail travel made easy" leaflet, available from Travel Centres and staffed stations. It takes up to 2 weeks to obtain a new or renewed railcard, so applications should be made ahead of any planned journeys. A Disabled Persons Railcard application helpline is available on ☎ 0191 218 8103; Textphone: 0191 269 0304 or see Ⓦ www.disabledpersons-railcard.co.uk.

Cross-channel services

As an alternative to ferries or planes, the Channel Tunnel offers a useful means for some people to travel to continental Europe. Two services exist.:

Eurostar train services from London St Pancras International, Ebbsfleet and Ashford to Brussels, Lille and Paris offer reduced rates for passengers travelling in wheelchairs and also for a companion. As spaces are limited, they should be booked in advance on
☎ 0870 518 6186. Other assistance is available on request at check-in although people are asked to arrive as early as they can. Information is available on
Ⓦ www.eurostar.com

Eurotunnel operates vehicle-carrying shuttle trains through the tunnel between Folkestone and Calais. Drivers of cars containing disabled people are asked to make themselves known at check-in so that they can be loaded at the front of the shuttle. Only 5 vehicles carrying disabled passengers who may need assistance in the event of an emergency evacuation can be carried in any shuttle. The terminals are accessible and have toilets for disabled people. However there is no need for disabled people to get out of their vehicles if they do not wish to. Information is available from Eurotunnel Customer Relations Department ☎ 0800 0969 992. ⓦ www.eurotunnel.co.uk

Taxis

In London, all licensed taxis have to be able to carry a passenger in a standard wheelchair. Therefore all of the "London black cabs" manufactured since 1989 have had to have space to carry a passenger in a manual wheelchair and either carry or be equipped with a ramp. This has had an impact elsewhere, particularly large urban areas, although the licensing is in the hands of the local authority.

In some areas price concession systems are available to disabled people for use on journeys by taxis and/or private hire cars. This may be as part of a more general concession scheme or a separate system. On a local basis, other specialist taxi services may exist for disabled people.

www.traintaxi.co.uk is a database giving information on the availability of taxis at stations throughout Britain. It includes telephone numbers for up to 3 taxi companies for advanced bookings and those that are said to have accessible vehicles are indicated, although individual requirements should be checked before booking.

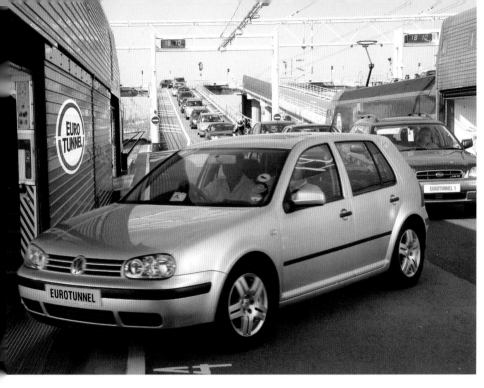
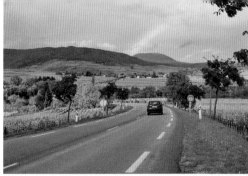
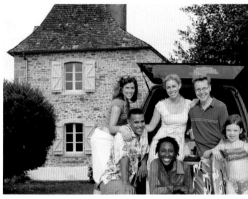

France, accessible to all...

...in just 35 minutes

- Stay in the comfort of your vehicle

- Disabled facilities in our Terminal

- Up to 3 departures per hour

- Price includes up to 9 passengers

Prices start from

£42

per car, each way
5 day return*

Book early for the best prices!

eurotunnel.com/radar

01303 28 25 55

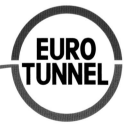

*Ticket must be purchased as part of a 5 day return. Subject to availability

FOLKESTONE - CALAIS

GEDESS 464253

THE MOTORISTS' NO.1 CHOICE FOR CROSSING THE CHANNEL

Trams and Underground Systems

Trams and other light rail systems have been developed over recent years in a number of places including Croydon, Greater Manchester, Nottingham, Sheffield and the West Midlands. These have all been fully designed to be usable by disabled people. Two earlier systems, the Tyne Wear Metro and the Docklands Light Railway in East London, are basically accessible to wheelchair users but they may need to be accompanied.

The older underground systems in London and the Glasgow Subway still provide only limited access for disabled passengers. In London new developments, such as the Jubilee Line extension between Westminster and Stratford, have been designed to be usable and a programme to create step-free routes to the platforms at almost 100 stations is underway together with other access improvements. Stations with platforms that can be reached without steps are indicated on Underground Maps published by Transport for London.

Travel Training

Some disabled people may need assistance and encouragement to make full and safe use of the growth of accessible public transport, particularly those for whom special transport has been provided. In some areas travel training is available to help disabled people use accessible buses and other forms of public transport independently.

A source of information is Coolmove, a network of people involved with independent travel training mainly of young people. Contact Don Walker, Independent Travel Co-ordinator, Hawkley Brook College, Kelvin Grove, Wigan WN3 6SP.
@ info@coolmove.org.uk Ⓦ www.coolmove.org.uk

RELATIONSHIPS AND LIFE EVENTS

Disabled people have relationships as deep and lasting as non-disabled people, making the same choices in sexual and personal relationships as anyone else.

Having an impairment does not stop you from enjoying your sexuality it may just mean rethinking your approach to sex and making practical adjustments. We all have sexual problems from time to time. There is lots of practical advice and peer support available. You should be able to access mainstream services via your GP and/or you may want to access services provided by disability organisations.

Brook
421 Highgate Studios, 53-79 Highgate Road, London NW5 1TL.
☎ 020 7284 6040.
@ admin@brookcentres.org.uk
Ⓦ www.brook.org.uk

Brook Advisory Centres provide confidential advice on sex and contraception for people aged up to 25. The Ask Brook confidential information and enquiry line for young people can be contacted on ☎ 0800 0185 023.

FPA
50 Featherstone Street, London EC1Y 8QU.
☎ 020 7608 5240.
Ⓦ www.fpa.org.uk

FPA, previously the Family Planning Association, works to improve the sexual health and reproductive rights of people throughout the UK. It has a wide range of publications and offers a training and consultancy service for professionals and community workers. The FPA Helpline, a confidential helpline for the public on all aspects of sexual and reproductive health is available on weekdays ☎ 0845 122 8690.

FPA has published a guide to legislation regarding sexual activity and people with learning disabilities including capacity to consent, intimate care, the use of sex workers and contraception. Learning Disabilities, Sex and the Law by Clare Fanstone and Sarah Andrews is available from FPA Direct on 0845 122 8600, price £13.99.

FPA Northern Ireland
3rd Floor, 67 Ascot House, 24-31 Shaftesbury Avenue, Belfast BT2 7DB.
☎ 0845 122 8687(helpline).

FPA Scotland
Unit 10, Firhill Business Centre, 76 Firhill Road, Glasgow G20 7BA.
☎ 0141 948 1179.

FPA Wales
Suite D1, Canton House, 435-451 Cowbridge Road East, Cardiff CF5 1JH.
☎ 029 2064 4034.

Outsiders Club

4S Leroy House, 435 Essex Road,
London N1 3QP.
☎ 020 7354 8291.
@ info@Outsiders.org.uk
Ⓦ www.outsiders.org.uk

Outsiders is for people who have
become isolated as a result of disability.
Members are offered the chance to
practice socialising and gain confidence.
Anyone over 16 may join and nobody is
turned away because of their physical
or social disability. Members receive a
magazine, membership list and a book
giving information on the problems
existing members have overcome.
Regular social gatherings are held in
central London and other gatherings are
arranged. Individual advice is available
by calling the Sex and Disability Helpline
on 0707 499 3527 or email: sexdis@
Outsiders.org.uk

Regard

BM Regard, London WC1N 3XX.
@ secretary@regard.org.uk
Ⓦ www.regard.org.uk

Regard is the national organisation of
Disabled Lesbians, Gay Men, Bisexuals
and Transgendered People. It aims to
raise awareness of disability issues
within the Lesbian, Gay, Bisexual and
Transgendered (LGBT) communities, and
to raise awareness of sexuality issues
within the disability communities. It
also works to combat social isolation
amongst its membership, and to
campaign on issues specifically affecting
disabled LGBT people.

Relate

Premier House, Caroline Court, Lakeside,
Doncaster DN4 5RA.
☎ 0300 100 1234.
@ enquiries@relate.org.uk
Ⓦ www.relate.org.uk

Relate is the largest organisation in the
country providing advice, relationship
counselling, sex therapy and other
forms of support. It operates from 600
locations in England, Wales and Northern
Ireland providing services face-to-face,
by telephone and over the internet.

In Scotland similar services are
provided by:
Relationships Scotland, 18 York Place,
Edinburgh EH1 3EP.
☎ 0845 119 6089.
Ⓦ www.relationships-scotland.org.uk

Respond

3rd Floor, 24-32 Stephenson Way,
London NW1 2HD.
☎ 020 7383 0700.
@ admin@respond.org.uk
Ⓦ www.respond.org.uk

Respond provides services to people with
learning disabilities who have experienced
abuse, bereavement or trauma as well
as to learning disabled perpetrators
of abuse and to parents with learning
disabilities. The services offered include
psychotherapy, risk assessment, training
and consultancy. A helpline is available on
0808 808 0700.

A number of other national disability organisations provide information and advice on sex and relationships:

❯ **The Spinal Injuries Association** has published a book called "Sex Matters"; it can give advice for anyone who's experiencing difficulties with their sex life. You can call its helpline on 0800 980 0501 for a booklet or to speak to someone directly. Ⓦ www.spinal.co.uk.

❯ If you're affected by Multiple Sclerosis (MS), **The Multiple Sclerosis Society** has a section of its website devoted to sex, intimacy and relationships. Helpline 0808 800 8000. @ helpline@mssociety.org.uk. Ⓦ www.mssociety.org.uk

❯ **Arthritis Care** has produced a booklet titled: "Relationships, Intimacy and Arthritis". Ⓦ www.arthritiscare.org.uk

❯ **The Stroke Association** has published a factsheet on "Sex after stroke" available from their website www.stroke.org.uk. Stroke helpline 0845 3033 100.

❯ **Warrington Disability Partnership** has produced a Relationships & Sex Matters Disability Information File. Ⓦ www.disabilitypartnership.org.uk @ info@disabilitypartnership.org.uk ☎ 01925 240064.

Parenting

The right to marry and to found a family is a basic human right. Social care and health services should support this right. When you have an assessment of your social care needs (see Independent Living Section) this should cover any support you need to carry out your parenting responsibilities. If you are a parent-to-be, you can let social services team know about your situation before your baby is born to help them plan your support.

The Disability Discrimination Act protects disabled parents (and prospective parents) against unlawful discrimination. For example classes for parents-to-be should make 'reasonable adjustments' to make them accessible; you should not be denied fertility treatment because of your disability; and you can't be treated unfairly by adoption and fostering services. Childcare providers and schools also have duties under the DDA to make their services accessible to you.

Deaf Parenting UK
SMS: 07789 027186.
@ info@deafparent.org.uk
Ⓦ www.deafparent.org.uk

DPUK is open to all Deaf adults with responsibility for children. It works to empower and support Deaf parents and to improve access to information and services.

Disability Pregnancy & Parenthood International

Unit F9, 89-93 Fonthill Road,
London N4 3JH.
☎ 0800 018 4730.
Textphone: 0800 018 9949.
@ info@dppi.org.uk Ⓦ www.dppi.org.uk

DPPI, a charity controlled by disabled parents, promotes better awareness and support for disabled people during and after pregnancy and as parents. It has a number of publications, offers training for health and social work professionals and provides a UK information service.

Disabled Parents Network
81 Melton Road, West Bridgford,
Nottingham NG2 8EN.
☎ 0870 241 0450.
@ information@disabledparentsnetwork.org.uk
Ⓦ www.disabledparentsnetwork.org.uk

The DPN is a membership organisation of and for disabled parents. It operates a peer support/contact register, issues a newsletter and runs a helpline operated by disabled parent volunteers. It campaigns for improved services for disabled parents, collaborates on research projects and provides training sessions for professionals and other interested organisations. A Helpline is available on ☎ 0300 3300 639.

> Advice to nurses and midwifes on improving the level of care for disabled women who are pregnant is contained in the Pregnancy and Disability booklet issued by the Royal College of Nursing.

Violence & Abuse

Sexual violence, financial abuse and other forms of violence and abuse – including neglect - are all crimes, whether they happen in your home, in the community or in institutions. There are lots of organisations who can support you. If you or someone you know is facing violence, abuse or neglect it's vital to tell your local council, the police or otherwise seek support.

Social and health care providers have to carry out criminal record checks and other checks on staff to make sure they have not abused, neglected or harmed people they have provided care and support to. If you are employing your own PA you have the right to these checks. Contact your local authority.

The Disability Equality Duty (see Discrimination section) places duties on local authorities, the police and housing associations to take positive action to stamp out harassment against disabled people.

Any crime that involves an element of hostility to someone because of their disability is a 'disability hate crime' and can attract a stiffer sentence – in some areas there are 'third party reporting sites' where you can go to report disability hate crime, otherwise you can report it to the police. Your local council and local disability organisation should be able to provide further information or contact RADAR or Scope.

Action on Elder Abuse

Astral House, 1268 London Road,
Norbury, London SW16 4ER.
☎ 020 8765 7000.
@ enquiries@elderabuse.org.uk
Ⓦ www.elderabuse.org.uk

Action on Elder Abuse works in UK and Ireland to protect and prevent the abuse of vulnerable older adults. A Helpline is available on 0808 808 8141

Victim Support

☎ 0845 303 0900.
Ⓦ www.victimsupport.org.uk

Victim Support is the independent charity which helps people cope with the effects of crime. It provides free and confidential support and information to help you deal with your experience.

Voice UK

☎ 0845 122 8695.
Textphone 07797 800 642.
Ⓦ www.voiceuk.org.uk

Voice UK is a national charity supporting people with learning disabilities and other vulnerable people who have experienced crime or abuse. It provides a telephone helpline which is attended from 9am to 5pm Monday to Friday.

WITNESS

32-36 Loman Street, London SE1 0EH.
☎ 020 7922 7799
@ info@professionalboundaries.org.uk
Ⓦ www.safeboundaries.org.uk

WITNESS works with people reporting abuse by doctors, nurses, complementary therapists, counsellors and other professionals. It also carries out research on professional abuse and offers training on professional boundaries and abuse issues. As well as the people directly affected, friends, family, professionals and anyone who is concerned that abuse may be happening and needs to talk through their options can contact a Helpline on 0845 4500 300.

Women's Aid

Helpline (24 hours) 0808 200 0247.
Ⓦ www.womensaid.org.uk

Women's Aid is the key national charity working to end domestic violence against women and children. It supports a network of over 500 domestic and sexual violence services across the UK.

Other Important Life Events

Child Bereavement Charity

Aston House, West Wycombe,
High Wycombe HP14 3AG.
☎ 01494 446648.
@ enquiries@childbereavement.org.uk
Ⓦ www.childbereavement.org.uk

CBC provides support, information and training to all involved both when a child dies or is bereaved of someone important in their lives.

Cruse Bereavement Care

PO Box 800, Richmond, Surrey TW9 1RG.

☎ 020 8939 9530.

@ info@cruse.org.uk

Ⓦ www.crusebereavementcare.org.uk

Cruse Bereavement Care Northern Ireland

Piney Ridge, Knockbracken Healthcare Park, Saintfield Road. Belfast BT8 8BH.

☎ 028 9079 2419.

Cruse Bereavement Care Scotland

Riverview House, Friarton Road, Perth PH2 8DF.

☎ 01738 444178.

Ⓦ www.crusescotland.org.uk

Cruse Bereavement Care Cymru

Ty Energlyn, Heol Las, Caerphilly CF83 2TT.

☎ 029 2088 6913.

Cruse is a charity providing advice, counselling and information on practical matters for anyone bereaved. It has 134 branches and 5500 volunteers across the UK and offers training and publications to those working with bereaved people. There is a national telephone helpline on 0844 477 9400.

WORK

Employment is crucial for people living with ill-health, injury or disability. It's the chance to earn an income, to have a role, colleagues, social networks and the chance to progress. For anyone, finding and obtaining a sustainable job - and a career - that suits their skills, abilities and aspirations is no easy task and often disabled people find it harder than most. But there are supports available. There are also legal rights – you can negotiate for adjustments at work that can help and you can challenge discrimination if it occurs. Difficulties in securing employment are often due to lack of disability-awareness or confidence on the part of employers and to the lack of knowledge of the support systems that are available.

Anyone on Incapacity Benefit or Employment and Support Allowance (see Benefits section) is now provided with a tailored package of back to work support. Along with this has come greater 'conditionality', for example requirements to take part in work-focused interviews. Integration of support to get skills as well as employment is planned. Government is also taking action to improve employment opportunities for people with mental health problems, who have particularly low employment rates.

Employment Rights

The Disability Discrimination Act makes discrimination unlawful against 'disabled people'. This includes people with a wide range of mental and physical impairments/health conditions, from HIV and cancer to depression and dementia, as well as sensory, learning and physical impairments. You are covered if your impairment has a substantial adverse effect on day to day activities and is, or is expected to be, long-term i.e. at least a year (whether continuous or intermittent). See the Discrimination section for fuller details of who is covered.

Under the Disability Discrimination Act it is unlawful for an employer to discriminate against a disabled person and there are five types of employment discrimination:-

❯ Direct discrimination – for example an employer says they simply won't employ someone with a mental health problem

❯ Failure to make reasonable adjustments – see below

❯ Disability-related discrimination – the reason is linked to the disability but is not the disability itself, e.g. taking time off work (note this is the only type of discrimination that can be justified and the employer must have a 'material and substantial' reason).

❯ Victimisation – e.g. if you are treated unfairly because you help a disabled person bring a complaint under the DDA

❯ Harassment

Employers cannot discriminate in relation to:

❯ Recruitment

❯ Terms and Conditions

❯ Redundancy, redeployment and dismissal

The scope of employment covered by the Act has been expanded by regulations issued since 1995 and now covers virtually all fields of activity by virtually all employers.

Employers have a duty to make reasonable adjustments to the workplace or to the way in which the work is carried out so that a disabled employee is not placed at a substantial disadvantage when compared with one who is not disabled. Such adjustments will depend on the job, the individual and the impairment but may include:

❯ Changed working hours or shift patterns, for instance to avoid rush hour travel or to ensure shifts fit in with medication regimes

❯ More regular breaks for someone who needs to take medication or to drink regularly because of medication effects

❯ Time off for medical appointments (e.g. dialysis, counselling), that can be made up at other times

❯ Carrying out physical alterations to make the working environment accessible, from lowered desks to space to move around easily;

❯ ITC adaptations, e.g. screen readers or adapted keypads or simple spell checks

❯ Changed forms of management support or feedback – for example, a written task list for someone with a difficulty in sequencing

❯ Reallocating any non-essential tasks to another employee if a disabled person finds them difficult;

❯ Redeployment to a suitable alternative post;

❯ Acquiring or modifying equipment;

❯ Providing a reader or interpreter.

You may want to find out what others have found useful, so you can put in place your own 'reasonable adjustment' (many people make their own without even talking to the employer); or so you can discuss the issue with your manager from a position of knowledge. If you know what others have done and you understand what your employer may be able to do, you are more likely to be presenting a 'solution' to the employer, which may make it easier for them to understand and potentially agree. See RADAR's Doing Work Differently publication for examples from other disabled people.

If your employer discriminates against you or is not willing to make the adjustments you need, then you have a range of options. You should get advice about your DDA rights – try the Equality and Human Rights Commission/Equality Commission for Northern Ireland Helplines, ask a trade union official or a disability advocacy organisation.

First try raising an informal grievance – i.e. raise the issue with your line manager or Human Resources, ideally put forward practical suggestions to put things right. If that doesn't work you should put in a formal written grievance. Only if all this does not work should you consider putting in a complaint to the Employment Tribunal. This must be done within 3 months of the alleged discrimination (if you are required to use a grievance or disciplinary procedure first you have an extra 3 months). Seek advice and also seek support – the experience of taking a case to a tribunal can be stressful. A trade union official, a friend, an advocate may be able to support you.

Your tribunal complaint will usually be copied to the Advisory, Conciliation and Arbitration Service (ACAS). It will try to help you and the employer reach a satisfactory settlement. This can result in constructive resolutions.

Where an Employment Tribunal upholds a complaint of discrimination because of disability it can:

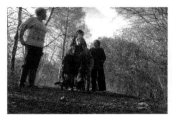
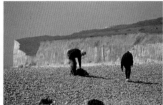
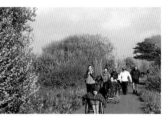

Natural England is an independent public body whose purpose is to protect and improve England's natural environment and encourage people to enjoy and get involved in their surroundings. We promote access, recreation and well-being and ensure natural resources are managed so they can be enjoyed now and by future generations.

In all our work we strive to ensure that the natural world is accessible to all and are committed to establishing a diverse and inclusive workforce. Your ability is what we are interested in, whether you want to apply for advertised roles or to volunteer your time and skills as part of our extensive volunteering programme. Our roles are as diverse as our people - from communications experts, environmental scientists, bat workers, business managers, to IT specialists. We welcome applications from people with disabilities and recruit through fair and open competition to all our posts.

If you think your skills could help Natural England conserve the natural environment, find out more from our website at www.naturalengland.org.uk.

★Stonewall
DIVERSITY CHAMPION

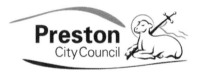

We are proud of our achievements in working towards equal opportunities in employment and access to services, helping make England's newest city a better place to live, work and visit.

To find out more about what's going on in our vibrant city and about job opportunities with Preston City Council visit our brand new website

www.preston.gov.uk

Work *Ability*

The Work Ability Programme is designed to help disabled people into employment within Kingston upon Hull City Council.

If you claim Incapacity Benefit, Income Support, Disability Living Allowance, Jobseeker's Allowance, Severe Disablement Allowance etc, this is a tailor-made voluntary scheme to help and support you to return to the world of work.

For an informal chat, Please contact 01482 612963

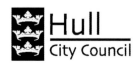

❯ say you have been discriminated against ('a declaration')

❯ recommend what your employer should do in the future to avoid discrimination ('a recommendation')

❯ award you money (compensation) for injury to feelings

❯ award you money for past and future loss of earnings.

The Equality and Human Rights Commission has a useful guide to the tribunal process.

ACAS
Brandon House, 180 Borough High Street, London SE1 1LW.
☎ 0845 747 4747.
Textphone: 0845 606 1600.
🖳 www.acas.org.uk

Equality and Human Rights Commission
See Discrimination section for contact details

Disability Champions @ Work is a project established by Amicus and TUC Education to recruit and train union members to help disabled people negotiate with employers to meet their needs and generally raise awareness of disability issues at work. There are over 750 Champions around the country, drawn from 31 unions, of whom 46% are disabled.
For further information see www.disabilitychampions.com

Employment Support

Jobcentre Plus combines employment services and employment related benefits for people of working age. Jobcentre Plus offers a range of services to people who are newly disabled and other disabled people who are having problems finding or keeping a job.

It can also give you information about the many employment support services in your area that may be provided by private or voluntary sector organisations (often under a contract from the Department for Work and Pensions).

A key feature of most of these services is the network of Disability Employment Advisers (DEAs) who can be contacted through local Jobcentre Plus offices.

DEAs can provide advice and information on job seeking, training and keeping a job as well as referring you to specialist services.

If you are concerned about losing your job for a reason relating to your disability or health condition a DEA can give you and your employer advice, and explore practical ways to help you keep your job.

Employment Assessment – This aims to find out how a disability or health condition affects the type of work or training that is needed. It will be carried out by a DEA, and possibly a work psychologist, and will result in an action plan. It will not affect your benefits. Travel expenses to take part in an employment assessment may be claimed.

DEAs can provide a **job-matching and referral** service to let you know about jobs that match your experience and skills. If you feel it's appropriate, the adviser may be able to approach the employer for you.

Specialist services they can refer you on to include:

Access to Work – Advice and practical support are available from an Access to Work Advisor to disabled people and their employers. This is backed up by a grant towards extra employment costs. The service is available if you are in a job, about to start a job or self-employed. The grant can cover communicator support at an interview (this is also available to unemployed people who need the service), a support worker, special aids and equipment, adaptations to premises or to existing equipment and help with additional costs of travel to work. Access to Work Advisers are based in 11 Regional teams covering England, Scotland and Wales. The contact details can be obtained from Jobcentre Plus Offices and are listed on www.jobcentreplus.com

Job Introduction Scheme – This scheme may be used when a disabled person wants to take up a job offer but where there are practical concerns about their ability to manage because of their disability. A JIS grant can be paid to the employer usually for the first 6 weeks of the employment. The JIS grant has to be agreed in advance and the job must be expected to last at least 6 months, including the grant period.

Work Preparation – A Work Preparation programme can last a few days or weeks depending on individual needs. It aims to help the participant by identifying the most suitable type of work, providing unpaid work experience with a local employer, providing new or up-dating old skills and building confidence. The programmes are run by outside providers usually in their own premises or the premises of a local employer. At the end of the programme a report is produced which can be discussed with the DEA.

WORKSTEP – The WORKSTEP programme provides supported jobs for disabled people with complex needs in relation to employment. Support to both employee and employer is tailored to individual requirements.

DEAs can also provide information on:

Pathways to Work – Pathways to Work programmes now operate throughout the country, providing individualised support to obtain employment for people receiving Employment Support Allowance or Incapacity Benefit or an equivalent benefit. Private organisations have been contracted to run Pathways to Work in many areas. For information contact Jobcentre Plus.

Training, skills and careers
(see also the Education and Skills section – lifelong learning)

The Government provides support to businesses with training and skills development for their employees through Train to Gain. If you're an employee looking to gain new skills, tell your employer about this new scheme. Your employer should contact a skills broker on **0800 015 55 45** to access advice and source high quality, vocational skills training
for staff.

In the future, a skills check will be offered at the same time as employment-related assessments, so people get integrated help with employment and skills. This may be particularly useful to disabled people, who have sometimes lost out on education and skills development and who may find relevant skills development useful during a recession, when jobs are scarce.

To develop your skills and career try a service called Nextstep. You get a personal Nextstep adviser who will talk with you in confidence to help you plan your future by linking your personal interests and skills to a job or career.

Your adviser will also help you:

❯ understand the job market

❯ search and apply for jobs

❯ find funding to support any learning

❯ develop your CV

❯ improve your interview and presentation skills

❯ by suggesting ways to progress in your current job

http://nextstep.direct.gov.uk

For advice on developing your educational potential, Skill offers advice and information. www.skill.org.uk

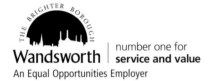

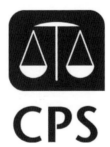

The Department for Work and Pensions still funds some residential training to help disabled adults who cannot get suitable training locally. It enables trainees to attend a residential training establishment providing individually tailored courses including work experience, training and guidance. Trainees receive an allowance with residential costs met by the Department. Courses, many leading to NVQs, are available at establishments throughout England most of which are also involved in Further Education although increasingly opportunities are being made available at local colleges to avoid separate provision. Applications are made through Disability Employment Advisers.

The programme is co-ordinated by The Residential Training Unit, Government Office for The North East, Citygate, Gallowgate, Newcastle upon Tyne NE1 4TD. ☎ 0191 202 3579. Textphone: 0191 202 3515. @ rtu@gone.gsi.gov.uk Ⓦ www.direct.gov.uk/disabledpeople

The providers that are part of the Residential Training programme for disabled adults are:

Doncaster College for the Deaf
Leger Way, Doncaster DN2 6AY.
☎ 01302 386700

Enham, Enham Alamein
Andover, Hampshire SP11 6JS.
☎ 01264 345800

Finchale Training College
Durham DH1 5RX.
☎ 0191 386 2634

Portland College
Nottingham Road, Mansfield, Nottinghamshire NG18 4TJ.
☎ 01623 499111

Queen Alexandra College
Court Oak Road, Harborne, Birmingham B17 9TG.
☎ 0121 428 5050

Queen Elizabeth's
Foundation Training College, Leatherhead Court, Leatherhead, Surrey KT22 0BN.
☎ 01372 841100

RNIB College Loughborough
Radmoor Road, Loughborough, Leicestershire LE11 3BS.
☎ 01509 611077

Royal National College for the Blind
College Road, Hereford HR1 1EB.
☎ 01432 265725.
Textphone: 01432 276532

St Loyes Foundation
Brittany House, New North Road, Exeter, Devon EX4 4EP.
☎ 01392 255428

Part-Time and Flexible Working

For some disabled people and carers, a full-time job with fixed, regular hours does not fit in to their needs. Part-time work may be one option. Job sharing is also becoming more popular and some organisations maintain a list of people who are willing to become job sharers. There are also ever increasing opportunities of working from home, using e-mail and the internet.

Disabled people may benefit from the greater general recognition by employers that their staff benefit from a better balance between their work and the rest of their life. One organisation that may be able to assist is:

Working Families

1-3 Berry Street, London EC1V 0AA.
☎ 020 7253 7243.
@ office@workingfamilies.org.uk
Ⓦ www.workingfamilies.org.uk.

Working Families supports and campaigns for working parents and carers. One of its projects is "Waving not Drowning" which supports parents who are trying to combine paid work and caring for disabled children. A free newsletter is published for parents and interested professionals and booklets provide information and highlight good practice for child-care professionals when working with clients who combine caring with paid employment.

Self-Employment

Disabled people have set up many successful businesses. Although it may seem daunting, self-employment or being part of a co-operative can offer a degree of flexibility and personal control that particularly suits some disabled people.

General help and advice on setting up a business and overcoming or avoiding problems can be obtained from Business Link. This is managed by the Department for Business, Enterprise & Regulatory

Reform and provides services on-line and through a network of local operators in England with similar services elsewhere in the UK. Contact:

Business Link

☎ 0845 600 9006.
Textphone: 0845 606 2666.
Ⓦ www.businesslink.gov.uk

Invest Northern Ireland

☎ 028 9023 9090.
Ⓦ www.investni.com

Business Gateway

☎ 0845 609 6611.
Ⓦ www.bgateway.com

Highlands & Islands Enterprise

☎ 0845 609 6611.
Ⓦ www.hiebusiness.co.uk

Flexible Support for Business

☎ 03000 6 03000.
Ⓦ www.business-support-wales.gov.uk

The Prince's Trust

18 Park Square East,
London NW1 4LH.
☎ 0800 842842.
Textphone: 020 7543 1374.
Ⓦ www.princes-trust.org.uk

Block 5, Jennymount Court,
North Derby Street,
Belfast BT15 3HN.
☎ 028 9074 5454.

1st Floor, The Guildhall, 57 Queen
Street, Glasgow G1 3EN.
☎ 0141 204 4409.

Baltic House, Mount Stuart Square,
Cardiff CF10 5FH.
☎ 029 2043 7000.

The Prince's Trust assists unemployed
or underemployed young people set up in
business with financial help and on-going
business advice.

Volunteering

Voluntary work can provide an opportunity to get in touch with the world of
work and a chance to learn new skills and meet people. Volunteers can offer their
time to help organisations in a wide variety of roles. Many areas have a Volunteer
Bureau where information on local opportunities can be obtained. Information
can be also be found on the national volunteering database www.do-it.org.uk.
Voluntary work should not affect benefits but if you have any doubts check with
a benefits advisor or the organisations listed below before taking on any regular
commitment. Further information on volunteering can be obtained from:

Volunteering England, Regents Wharf

8 All Saints Street, London N1 9RL.
☎ 0845 305 6979.
@ volunteering@volunteeringengland.org
Ⓦ www.volunteering.org.uk

Volunteer Development Agency Northern Ireland,

129 Ormeau Road, Belfast BT7 1SH.
☎ 028 9023 6100.
Ⓦ www.volunteering-ni.org

Volunteer Development Scotland

Stirling Enterprise Park, Stirling
FK7 7RP.
☎ 01786 479593.
Ⓦ www.vds.org.uk

Wales Council for Voluntary Action

Baltic House, Mount Stuart Square,
Cardiff Bay, Cardiff CF10 5FH.
☎ 029 2043 1700.
Textphone: 029 2043 1702.
Ⓦ www.wcva.org.uk

Community Service Volunteers

237 Pentonville Road, London N1 9NJ.
☎ 020 7278 6601.
@ information@csv.org.uk
Ⓦ www.csv.org.uk

CSV is Britain's largest volunteer
organisation and provides opportunities
for people with disabilities and learning
difficulties to take part in a number of
its projects.

Useful Organisations

Association of Disabled Professionals

BCM ADP, London WC1N 3XX.
☎ 01204 431638.
@ adp.admin@ntlworld.com
Ⓦ www.adp.org.uk

The ADP draws its members from disabled people working, or having worked, in the professions or in a managerial role. It has established the Disabled Entrepreneurs' Network to provide networking opportunities among self-employed disabled people and those setting up and running their own businesses.

British Association for Supported Employment

Unit 26 Severnside Trading Estate, Sudmeadow Road, Hempsted, Gloucester GL2 5HS.
☎ 08445 617445.
@ admin@base-uk.org
Ⓦ www.afse.org.uk

BASE supports agencies and staff providing supported employment. It represents around 200 organisations around the country providing them with information and training and encourages the development of new services.

Disabled Workers Co-operative

The Old Vicarage, Myddfai, Carmarthenshire SA20 0JE.
Ⓦ www.disabledworkers.org.uk

The Disabled Workers Co-operative has a database of skills and services offered by disabled workers. The information enables potential clients to get in touch with disabled service providers in their locality. Any disabled individual, sheltered workshop or organisation employing a significant number of disabled people can register free on the database, which is also free to use by visiting the website. The website also has e-jobs portal where disabled people looking for employment can browse for jobs and employers can post their vacancies free.

Employers' Forum on Disability

Nutmeg House, 60 Gainsford Street, London SE1 2NY.
☎ 020 7403 3020.
Textphone: 020 7403 0040.
Ⓦ www.efd.org.uk

The Employers Forum on Disability promotes and develops good practice among employers in the employment of disabled people and service to disabled customers. The Forum has around 400 members representing over 20% of the workforce and provides wide-ranging advice and information to them.

Enham

Enham Alamein, Andover SP11 6JS.
☎ 01264 345800.
Ⓦ www.enham.org.uk

From its base in Hampshire, Enham provides a wide range of employment and training services for disabled people.

Remploy

Stonecourt, Siskin Drive, Coventry CV3 4FJ.
☎ 0800 138 7656.
Textphone: 024 7651 5869
@ info@remploy.co.uk
Ⓦ www.remploy.co.uk

Remploy is the UK's leading provider of jobs for disabled people. The company partners some of the country's biggest companies to find jobs for disabled people. Remploy employs around 3,000 disabled people in its own manufacturing and services businesses and last year its employment services division found 6,500 jobs for people with a range of physical, sensory and mental disabilities in mainstream employment.

Shaw Trust

Fox Talbot House, Greenways Business Park, Chippenham SN15 1BN.
☎ 01225 716300.
Textphone: 0845 769 7288.
Ⓦ www.shaw-trust.org.uk

The Shaw Trust has grown to become one of the largest organisations providing training and employment support for disabled and disadvantaged people in Great Britain. It offers a wide range of training, employment preparation, work placements, help in moving from benefits to work and long term supported employment to meet the individual needs of disabled people.

Many other organisations, including some of the national disability specific organisations listed elsewhere in the book and those working locally, also provide employment related services and support.

USEFUL CONTACTS

General Disability Information

Advice Service Capability Scotland
11 Ellersly Road, Edinburgh EH12 6HY.
☎ 0131 313 5510.
Textphone: 0131 346 2529.
@ ascs@capability-scotland.org.uk
Ⓦ www.capability-scotland.org.uk

General advice on disability issues
as well as more specialist advice on
cerebral palsy is available from ASCS at
the above address.

Contact a Family
209-211 City Road, London EC1V 1JN.
☎ 020 7608 8700.
Textphone: 0808 808 3556.
@ helpline@cafamily.org.uk
Ⓦ www.cafamily.org.uk

Contact a Family offers information,
advice and support to families who care
for disabled children. It holds information
on over 1000 rare syndromes and
disorders and can put families in touch
with each other and support groups.
Information is also provided on a wide
range of issues including assessments,
benefits and education. There is a
network of Contact a Family offices
and representatives across the UK. A
Helpline is available, 10am-4pm Monday-
Friday and 5.30-7.30pm Mondays on
☎ 0808 808 3555.

www.direct.gov.uk/disabledpeople
Directgov is the government's consumer
website giving information on public
services with links to government
departments and agencies and a wide
range of other organisations.

Disability Action
Portside Business Park, 189 Airport
Road West, Belfast BT3 9ED.
☎ 028 9029 7880.
Textphone: 028 9029 7882.
@ information@disabilityaction.org
Ⓦ www.disabilityaction.org

The Northern Ireland pan-disability
organisation can provide information on
services for disabled people in Northern
Ireland.

Disability Wales/Anabledd Cymru
Bridge House, Caerphilly Business Park,
Van Road, Caerphilly CF83 3GW.
☎ 029 2088 7325.
@ info@disabilitywales.org
Ⓦ www.disabilitywales.org

Disability Wales is a national association
of disability groups in Wales promoting
rights, inclusion, equality and support of
all disabled people. It publishes leaflets
and provides an information service.

Equality and Human Rights Commission
See full listing in Discrimination section.

United Kingdom's Disabled People's Council
Litchurch Plaza, Litchurch Lane,
Derby DE24 8AA.
☎ 01332 295551.
Textphone: 01332 295581.
@ general@UKSDPC.org
Ⓦ www.bcodp.org.uk

UKDPC's members are organisations controlled by disabled people. Information on campaigns and a wide range of matters can be obtained through its website.

UPDATE
Hays Business Centre,
4 Hay Avenue, Edinburgh EH16 4AQ.
☎ 0131 669 1600.
@ info@update.org.uk   Ⓦ www.update.org.uk

UPDATE is Scotland's national disability information organisation. It provides a public helpline service on the above telephone number, although people may be referred to organisations that are more appropriate whether geographically or because they have more specialised knowledge.

Local Advice Services

Advice on services and support in obtaining them often needs to be obtained locally. A wide range of local organisations exists including those specifically related to disability and those offering a more general service.

Dial UK is the national organisation for the **DIAL Network** – a network of approximately 120 Disability Information and Advice Line services run by disabled people providing free, impartial and confidential information services for disabled people and their families and advisors mainly by telephone. Some also offer additional services. Information on local DIAL groups, but not individual advice, can be obtained from Dial UK, St Catherine's, Tickhill Road, Doncaster DN4 8QN.
☎ /Textphone: 01302 310123. @ informationenquiries@dialuk.org.uk
Ⓦ www.dialuk.info

Advocacy is taking action to help people who find themselves in a position where their ability to exercise choice or represent their own interests is limited, and to help them to say what they want, to secure their rights, to represent their interests and to obtain the services they need. Advocacy schemes can be national or local, concerned with specific clusters of needs or be more general. Information on local advocacy schemes is available from:

Action for Advocacy
PO Box 31856, Lorrimore Square,
London SE17 3XR.
☎ 020 7820 7868.
@ info@actionforadvocacy.org.uk
Ⓦ www.actionforadvocacy.org.uk

Scottish Independent Advocacy Alliance
Melrose House, 69a George Street,
Edinburgh EH2 2JG.
☎ 0131 260 5380.
Ⓦ www.siaa.org.uk

The Citizens Advice service helps people resolve legal, financial and other problems by providing free information and advice from over 3200 locations. Online advice, downloadable fact sheets and the location of Citizens Advice Bureaux are available on www.adviceguide.org.uk

Information on the services available from, and contact details for, individual Bureaux in England and Wales, but not advice, can be obtained from:

Citizens Advice
Myddelton House, 115-123 Pentonville Road, London N1 9LZ.
ⓦ www.citizensadvice.org.uk

For elsewhere in the UK contact:

Citizens Advice Northern Ireland
46 Donegall Pass, Belfast BT7 1BS.
ⓦ www.citizensadvice.co.uk

Citizens Advice Scotland
1st Floor, Spectrum House, 2 Powderhall Road, Edinburgh EH7 4GB.
ⓦ www.cas.org.uk

Specific Disabilities

There are many organisations concerned with specific conditions and impairments. While some are mainly concerned with research and/or medical treatment, many provide services, information and the opportunity for mutual support. The following is just a selection of relevant organisations.

Action for Blind People
14-16 Verney Road, London SE16 3DZ.
☎ 020 7635 4800.
@ info@actionforblindpeople.org.uk
ⓦ www.actionforblindpeople.org.uk

Action for Blind People offers services, particularly in the fields of employment, housing, holidays, sport and information to blind and partially sighted people of all ages. A Freephone Helpline is available on: ☎ 0800 915 4666.

ADDISS
PO Box 340, Edgware, Middlesex HA8 9HL.
☎ 020 8952 2800.
@ info@addiss.co.uk
ⓦ www.addiss.co.uk

ADDISS (Attention Deficit Disorder Information & Support Service) provides information and resources about attention deficit hyperactivity disorder to anyone who needs assistance through publications, a website and by telephone.

Afasic – Unlocking Speech and Language

1st Floor, 20 Bowling Green Lane, London EC1R 0BD.
☎ 020 7490 9410.
@ info@afasic.org.uk
Ⓦ www.afasic.org.uk

Afasic represents children and young adults with speech, language and communication impairments, working for their inclusion in society and supporting their parents and carers. Afasic provides children, young people, families and professionals with:

❯ Training, seminars and conferences

❯ Information sheets, newsletters and publications

❯ Support through local groups

❯ Expertise in developing good practice

❯ A telephone helpline service on
  ☎ 0845 355 5577

Elsewhere in the UK contact:

Afasic Scotland

Gemini Crescent, Dundee Technology Park, Dundee DD2 1TY.
☎ 01382 561891.

Afasic Cymru

Titan House, Cardiff Bay Business Centre, Lewis Road, Ocean Park, Cardiff CF24 5BS.
☎ 029 2046 5854.

Afasic Northern Ireland

Cranogue House, 19 Derrycourtney Road, Caledon, County Tyrone, Belfast BT68 4UF.
☎ 028 3756 9611.

Allergy UK

3 White Oak Square, London Road, Swanley, Kent BR8 7AG.
☎ 01322 619898.
@ info@allergyuk.org
Ⓦ www.allergyuk.org

Allergy UK aims to increase understanding of allergy, food intolerance and chemical sensitivity, to help people manage their allergies, to fund research and provide training in allergy for health care professionals. It provides leaflets, factsheets and operates a Helpline on the above number on weekdays from 9am-5pm.

Alzheimer's Society

Devon House, 58 St Katharine's Way, London E1W 1JX.
☎ 020 7423 3500.
@ enquiries@alzheimers.org.uk
Ⓦ www.alzheimers.org.uk

Information and support are provided for people with dementia and their families from the national office, through regional networks and a network of over 250 branches in England, Northern Ireland and Wales. Contact details on these local branches and information on the areas covered can be found on its website.
The Alzheimer's Society Dementia Helpline is available on ☎ 0845 300 0336.

Alzheimer Scotland

22 Drumsheugh Gardens, Edinburgh EH3 7RN.
☎ 0808 808 3000 (Helpline) or 0131 243 1453.
@ alzheimer@alzscot.org
Ⓦ www.alzscot.org

Alzheimer Scotland provides care, understanding and support for people with dementia and their carers with practical services at over 60 sites throughout Scotland.

Arthritis Care

18 Stephenson Way, London NW1 2HD.
☎ 020 7380 6500.
@ info@arthritis.org.uk
Ⓦ www.arthritiscare.org.uk

Unit 4 McCune Building, 1 Shore Road,
Belfast BT15 3PG.
☎ 028 9078 2940.

Unit 25A, Anniesland Business Park,
Glasgow G13 1EU.
☎ 0141 954 7776.

Electric House, Castle Street,
Newcastle Emlyn, Carmarthenshire
SA38 9AF.
☎ 0845 241 9676.

Arthritis Care campaigns both directly
and through its branch network as well
as providing information and services for
people with arthritis.

Arthritis Research Campaign

Copeman House, St Mary's Court, St
Mary's Gate, Chesterfield S41 7TD.
☎ 0870 850 5000.
@ info@arc.org.uk
Ⓦ www.arc.org.uk

In addition to funding medical research,
arc publishes a wide range of free advice
booklets and information sheets about
all the different types of arthritis and
musculoskeletal conditions covering
drugs, symptoms and self-management.

ASBAH – Association for Spina Bifida & Hydrocephalus

42 Park Road, Peterborough PE1 2UQ.
☎ 01733 421309.
@ helpline@asbah.org
Ⓦ www.asbah.org

ASBAH provides information and advice
about spina bifida and hydrocephalus
to individuals, families and carers with
services targeted to:

❯ support for parents before and around
   the birth of their baby, or diagnosis of
   the disability

❯ support to the child and family on
   educational matters

❯ specialised information and help on
   health matters

❯ helping young people get services to
   move towards control of their lives

❯ responding to the needs of adults
   with spina bifida and hydrocephalus.

It has a network of advisers throughout
England, Wales and Northern Ireland
and specialist advisers in the fields
of education, medical matters and
continence management. There are
also local groups in many areas. A
Helpline is available on weekdays on
0845 450 7755.

In Scotland contact:
Scottish Spina Bifida Association,
The Dan Young Building, 6 Craighalbert
Way, Cumbernauld G68 0LS.
☎ 01236 794500,
Helpline 0845 911 1112.
Ⓦ www.ssba.org.uk

Asthma UK

Summit House, 70 Wilson Street,
London EC2A 2DB.
☎ 020 7786 4900.
@ info@asthma.org.uk
Ⓦ www.asthma.org.uk

The Mount, 2 Woodstock Link,
Belfast BT6 8DD.
☎ 02890 737290.

4 Queen Street, Edinburgh EH2 1JE.
☎ 0131 226 2544.

3rd Floor, Eastgate House, 34-43
Newport Road, Cardiff CF24 0AB.
☎ 02920 435 400.

Asthma UK works to improve the
health and well being of people whose
lives are affected by asthma. It works
with people with asthma, professionals
and researchers to develop and share
expertise to help people increase their
understanding and reduce the effect of
asthma on their lives. Asthma nurse
specialists provide information on an
Adviceline ☎ 0800 121 6244 (Monday-
Friday 9am-5pm).

Ataxia UK

Lincoln House, Kennington Park, 1-3
Brixton Road, London SW9 6DE.
☎ 020 7582 1444.
@ enquiries@ataxia.org.uk
Ⓦ www.ataxia.org.uk

Ataxia UK is concerned with most forms
of cerebellar ataxia and helps people
throughout the UK live with the effects
of ataxia through information leaflets,
a quarterly magazine, conferences, a
network of branches and self-help groups
as well as information on its website. It
also funds medical research. A helpline is
available on 0845 644 0606.

BackCare – National Back Pain Association

16 Elmtree Road, Teddington, Middlesex
TW11 8ST.
☎ 020 8977 5474.
@ info@backcare.org.uk
Ⓦ www.backcare.org.uk

BackCare, a national charity, provides
independent information on the
causes, treatments and management
of back pain. It can supply a range of
publications, has a network of local
branches and operates a telephone
helpline on
☎ 0845 130 2704.

beat

103 Prince of Wales Road, Norwich
NR1 1DW.
☎ 0870 770 3256.
@ info@b-eat.co.uk
Ⓦ www.b-eat.co.uk

Beat, previously the Eating Disorders
Association, supports and informs
people affected by eating disorders, such
as anorexia, bulimia and binge eating,
as well as their families and friends.
It has adult and youth helplines, email
services and a searchable database of
treatment services. It runs a network
of support groups and offer training for
professionals. Helplines available:
0845 634 1414, beat Youthline on
0845 634 7650.

Bladder & Bowel Foundation

SATRA Innovation Park, Rockingham
Road, Kettering NN16 9JH.
☎ 0870 770 3246.
@ info@bladderandbowelfoundation.org
Ⓦ www.bladderandbowelfoundation.org

B&BF is a UK advocacy charity which campaigns for people with bowel and bladder control problems. It provides user-friendly booklets and a magazine and offers on-line support and a confidential telephone service giving information on local Continence Advisors. It also runs the annual Continence Awareness Week.

British Deaf Association

10th Floor, Coventry Point, Market Way, Coventry CV1 1EA.
☎ 02476 550936. Textphone: 02476 550393. @ midlands@bda.org.uk
Ⓦ www.bda.org.uk

Unit 19c, Weavers Court, Linfield Road, Belfast BT12 5GH.
☎ 028 9043 7480.
Textphone: 028 9043 7486.

Central Chambers, Suite 58, 93 Hope Street, Glasgow G2 6LD.
☎/Textphone: 0141 248 5554.

British Sign Language Cultural Centre, 47 Newport Road, Cardiff CF24 0AD.
☎ 0845 130 2851.
Textphone: 0845 130 2853.

The BDA campaigns for the rights and opportunities of those who use sign language. It runs an information and advice service, employs youth workers and can offer counselling in British Sign Language to deaf people.

British Dyslexia Association

Unit 8, Bracknell Beeches, Old Bracknell Lane, Bracknell RG12 7BW.
☎ 0845 251 9003. (Helpline), 0845 251 9002. @ admin@bdadyslexia.org.uk
Ⓦ www.bdadyslexia.org.uk

The British Dyslexia Association campaigns to raise awareness and understanding of dyslexia and the needs of dyslexic people and those they are in contact with.

British Heart Foundation

Greater London House, 180 Hampstead Road, London NW1 7AW.
☎ 020 7554 0000.
Ⓦ www.bhf.org.uk

The BHF provides information and sponsors 300 support groups around the country. An information and helpline is available on 0300 333 1333.

British Kidney Patient Association

Bordon, Hants GU35 9JZ.
☎ 01420 472021/2.
@ info@britishkidney-pa.co.uk
Ⓦ www.britishkidney-pa.co.uk

The BKPA provides information and financial support to kidney patients and their families including help with getting a holiday. Applications for grants should be made through a renal social worker.

British Lung Foundation

73-75 Goswell Road, London EC1V 7ER.
☎ 020 7688 5555.
@ enquiries@blf-uk.org
Ⓦ www.lunguk.org

The British Lung Foundation:

❯ supports people affected by lung disease, including through the nationwide network of Breathe Easy support groups;

❯ helps people understand their condition by providing clear information on paper, on the web and on the telephone helpline 0845 850 5020;

❯ works for positive change in lung health by campaigning, raising awareness and funding research.

A helpline is available on ☎ 0845 850 5020 (Monday-Friday 10am-6pm)

British Polio Fellowship

Eagle Office Centre, The Runway, South Ruislip HA4 6SE.
☎ 0800 018 0586.
@ info@britishpolio.org.uk
Ⓦ www.britishpolio.org.uk

The Polio Fellowship provides support, information and advice to people who have had polio, their families and anyone wanting more information about polio or Post Polio Syndrome living in the UK. The Fellowship is the largest national charity for people with polio and has a network of local branches and groups. It produces a bi-monthly magazine and offers information, grants, welfare services and a holiday programme, including a bungalow in Somerset. It also carries out campaigning and fundraising activities.

The British Stammering Association

15 Old Ford Road, London E2 9PJ.
☎ 020 8983 1003.
@ info@stammering.org
Ⓦ www.stammering.org

The Association provides information and support to people concerned about stammering through a telephone helpline on 0845 603 2001, an email service and its website. It has a library and shop selling specialist items. There are also local self-help and email groups offering activities and contacts for members.

Brittle Bone Society

Grant-Paterson House, 30 Guthrie Street, Dundee DD1 5BS.
☎ 01382 204446.
@ bbs@brittlebone.org
Ⓦ www.brittlebone.org

The Brittle Bone Society is a national support group for people with 'brittle bone disease' or Osteogenesis Imperfecta. It can provide advice to parents and some specialist equipment on loan. An advice helpline is available on 0800 0282 459.

CancerHelp UK

☎ 0808 800 4040.
Ⓦ www.cancerhelp.org.uk

Cancer Help UK is the information service on cancer and cancer services of Cancer Research UK. All web pages are written so that they can be endorsed by the Plain English Campaign. Specialist cancer nurses staff the helpline.

Changing Faces

Changing Faces Centre, 33-37 University Street, London WC1E 6JN.
☎ 0845 450 0275.
@ info@changingfaces.org.uk
Ⓦ www.changingfaces.org.uk

Changing Faces provides confidential support and advice to people with a visible difference or disfigurement to the face and their families and friends. Training and consultancy is offered to employers and professionals in health, care and education.

Coeliac UK

Suites A-D Octagon Court, High Wycombe HP11 2HS.
☎ 01494 437278.
Ⓦ www.coeliac.org.uk

Coeliac UK provides an information service and support through local groups for people affected by coeliac disease and intolerance to gluten. It produces a range of publications and factsheets on dietary and other issues. A helpline is available on 0870 444 8804.

Cystic Fibrosis Trust

11 London Road, Bromley BR1 1BY.
☎ 020 8464 7211.
@ enquiries@cftrust.org.uk
Ⓦ www.cftrust.org.uk

The Cystic Fibrosis Trust funds research to treat and cure Cystic Fibrosis (CF) and aims to ensure appropriate care and support for people with CF. It issues a variety of publications and provides a helpline service for advice and support on any aspect of CF. Helpline available on 0845 859 1000

Cystitis & Overactive Bladder Foundation

946 Bristol Road South, Northfield, Birmingham B31 2LQ.
☎ 0121 476 1222.
@ info@cobfoundation.org
Ⓦ www.cobfoundation.org

The COB Foundation is a membership organisation providing information and support for people with cystitis and other overactive bladder conditions and their families. It has a quarterly newsletter as well as local support groups. Education materials are provided for patients as well as professionals and research is monitored.

Deafblind UK

National Centre for Deafblindness, John and Lucille van Geest Place, Cygnet Road, Hampton, Peterborough PE7 8FD.
☎/Textphone 01733 358100.
@ info@deafblind.org.uk
Ⓦ www.deafblind.org.uk

Deafblind UK offers comprehensive services to deafblind people including a 24-hour Helpline on 0800 132320, training in communication, IT Training, assessment & rehabilitation, counselling, independent living accommodation, holidays/rallies and publications in large print, Braille, Moon and on audio-tape. Deafblind UK has regional staff throughout the UK, membership support workers and volunteers who help to identify deafblind people in the community, pinpoint their needs and ensure they are addressed.

In Scotland contact:
Deafblind Scotland, 21 Alexandra Avenue, Lenzie, Glasgow G66 5BG.
☎/Textphone: 0141 777 6111.
@ info@deafblindscotland.org.uk
Ⓦ www.deafblindscotland.org.uk

DeafPLUS

1st Floor, Trinity Centre, Key Close, London E1 4HG.
☎ 020 7790 6147. @ info@deafplus.org
Ⓦ www.deafplus.org

The aim of deafPLUS, is to develop innovative schemes with deaf and hearing people enabling them to improve their quality of life through contact, information and training. Services include a mobile advice service.

DebRA

13 Wellington Business Park, Dukes Ride, Crowthorne, Berkshire RG45 6LS.
☎ 01344 771961.
@ deb2ra@debra.org.uk
Ⓦ www.debra.org.uk

DebRA provides support for people with the skin blistering condition, epidermolysis bullosa, and researches treatments. Specialist nurses and social workers are employed to support parents and give advice. It publishes a range of literature and funds research.

Diabetes UK

Macleod House, 10 Parkway, London NW1 7AA.
☎ 020 7424 1000.
@ info@diabetes.org.uk
Ⓦ www.diabetes.org.uk

Diabetes UK campaigns for the rights of people with diabetes and is committed to providing support to them. A range of publications and local as well as national services are provided including family support weekends and children's support holidays. Advice and information is available on the Careline 0845 120 2960.

DIAL House Chester – Disability Services (Advice and Information, Café, Shopmobility)

DIAL House, Hamilton Place, Chester, CH1 2BH
☎ 01244 345655
@ contactus@dialhousechester.org.uk
Ⓦ www.dialhousechester.org.uk

Different Strokes

9 Canon Harnett Court, Wolverton Mill, Milton Keynes MK12 5NF.
☎ 0845 130 7172.
@ info@differentstrokes.co.uk
Ⓦ www.differentstrokes.co.uk

Different Strokes was established by and for younger stroke survivors of working age, to provide appropriate support and information. It provides information packs, a counselling service and a helpline giving access to advice and information. Its website includes a heavily used message board where members exchange information and support and share their own experiences of stroke.

Down's Syndrome Association

Langdon Down Centre, 2A Langdon Park, Teddington TW11 9PS.
☎ 0845 230 0372.
@ info@downs-syndrome.org.uk
Ⓦ www.downs-syndrome.org.uk

The Down's Syndrome Association provides information and support to people with Down's syndrome, their families and carers as well as being a resource for professionals. The Association also strives to improve knowledge of the condition and champions the rights of people with Down's syndrome.

Duchenne Family Support Group

78 York Street, London W1H 1DP.
☎ 0870 241 1857.
@ info@dfsg.org.uk   Ⓦ www.dfsg.org.uk

DFSG brings families affected by Duchenne muscular dystrophy together for mutual support, sharing of information and social activities. It organises holidays, workshops, an annual conference and offer supports on a helpline
☎ 0800 121 4518.

The Dyspraxia Foundation

8 West Alley, Hitchin, Hertfordshire SG5 1EG.
☎ 01462 455016.
@ dyspraxia@dyspraxiafoundation.org.uk
Ⓦ www.dyspraxiafoundation.org.uk

The Dyspraxia Foundation is a resource for children, teenagers and adults who have dyspraxia, their parents and families and for teachers and other professionals working with them. It has a number of local support groups and also provides information in publications, through conferences, its website and on the Helpline 01462 454986.

The Ear Foundation

Marjorie Sherman House, 83 Sherwin Road, Nottingham NG7 2FB.
☎ 0115 942 1985.
Ⓦ www.earfoundation.org.uk

The Ear Foundation supports and provides activities, courses and resources for deaf children, young people and adults with cochlear implants, their families and supporting professionals.

Epilepsy Action
New Anstey House, Gate Way Drive, Yeadon, Leeds LS19 7XY.
☎ 0113 210 8880.
@ helpline@epilepsy.org.uk
Ⓦ www.epilepsy.org.uk

Epilepsy Action provides services and information for anyone in the UK with an interest in epilepsy. A wide range of leaflets and other publications are available by post or on its website. A password protected online community is also available at www.forum4e.com. The Epilepsy Helpline can be contacted on 0808 800 5050.

In Scotland contact:

Epilepsy Scotland
48 Govan Road, Glasgow G51 1JL.
☎ 0808 800 2200 (Helpline), 0141 427 4911. @ enquiries@epilepsyscotland. org.uk
Ⓦ www.epilepsyscotland.org.uk

ERIC (Education & Resources for Improving Childhood Continence)
36 Old School House, Britannia Road, Kingswood, Bristol BS15 8DB.
☎ 0117 960 3060.
@ info@eric.org.uk
Ⓦ www.eric.org.uk or www.trusteric.org (for young people)

ERIC provides information and support to children, teenagers, parents and professionals on all aspects of childhood continence. It sells a range of products to help manage childhood continence problems through www.ericshop.org. uk. For a free catalogue, call 0117 301 2101. ERIC is campaigning to achieve better toilets and also to improve the provision of drinking water in schools. A helpline for information and support is available Monday-Friday 10am-4pm on 0845 370 8008.

For Dementia
6 Camden High Street, London NW1 0JH.
☎ 020 7874 7210.
@ info@fordementia.org.uk
Ⓦ www.fordementia.org.uk

For Dementia runs training courses for those caring for people with dementia and has a network of specialist admiral nurses working in the community with families affected by dementia. A helpline, Admiral Nursing Direct, is available on 0845 257 9406.

Haemophilia Society
1st Floor, Petersham House, 57a Hatton Garden, London EC1N 8JG.
☎ 020 7831 1020.
@ info@haemophilia.org.uk
Ⓦ www.haemophilia.org.uk

The Haemophilia Society aims to ensure all people with haemophilia and related bleeding disorders receive the best possible care, treatment and support. Particular attention is paid to the needs of children, young people, their families and women with bleeding disorders. It has 16 local groups and offers a forum as well as a Helpline on 0800 018 6068.

Headway – The Brain Injury Association
7 King Edward Court, King Edward Street, Nottingham NG1 1EW.
☎ 0115 924 0800.
Textphone: 0115 950 7852.
@ helpline@headway.org.uk
Ⓦ www.headway.org.uk

Headway supports the interests of people living with a brain injury, their families and carers. It has over 110 local groups and branches providing mutual support for people with brain injury and their carers and other services. A Helpline is available on 0808 800 2244.

Hearing Concern LINK

19 Hartfield Road, Eastbourne, East Sussex BN21 2AR.
☎ 01323 638230.
Textphone: 01323 739998.
@ helpdesk@hearingconcernlink.org
Ⓦ www.hearingconcernlink.org

Hearing Concern LINK provides advice, information and support to people with hearing loss, promotes communication access and raises public and professional awareness of the issues associated with hearing loss.

Hemihelp

Camelford House, 89 Albert Embankment, London SE1 7TP.
☎ 0845 120 3713 or
Helpline 0845 123 2372.
@ support@hemihelp.org.uk
Ⓦ www.hemihelp.org.uk

Hemihelp is a membership organisation offering advice and support to the families of children and young people with hemiplegia. It provides a telephone and email helpline service, an online message board, publishes leaflets, a quarterly newsletter and a book for children, holds activities for children with hemiplegia and organises conferences and workshops for parents and professionals.

Huntington's Disease Association

Neurosupport Centre, Liverpool L3 8LR.
☎ 0151 298 3298.
@ info@hda.org.uk
Ⓦ www.hda.org.uk

As well as supporting research into treatment for Huntington's Disease, the Association provides a central information and advice service, a network of Regional Care Advisers and has local groups throughout the country.

In Scotland similar services are provided by:

Scottish Huntington's Association

Suite 135, St James Business Centre, Linwood Road, Paisley PA3 3AT.
☎ 0141 848 0308.
Ⓦ www.hdscotland.org

Insulin Dependent Diabetes Trust

PO Box 294, Northampton NN1 4XS.
☎ 01604 622837.
@ enquiries@iddtinternational.org
Ⓦ www.iddtinternational.org

IDDT is an organisation run by people with diabetes and their relatives that campaigns for informed choice of treatment and the continued availability of animal insulin. It publishes a range of information leaflets and a quarterly newsletter.

Jennifer Trust for Spinal Muscular Atrophy

Elta House, Birmingham Road, Stratford upon Avon, Warwickshire CV37 0AQ.
☎ 01789 267520.
@ Jennifer@jtsma.org.uk
Ⓦ www.jtsma.org.uk

The Jennifer Trust supports and provides information for children and adults with spinal muscular atrophy and their families. A helpline is available on 0800 975 3100.

Limbless Association

Queen Mary's Hospital, Roehampton Lane, London SW15 5PN.
☎ 020 8788 1777.
@ enquiries@limbless-association.org
Ⓦ www.limbless-association.org

The Limbless Association promotes the interests of limbless people of all ages around the country. Its programmes include a volunteer visitor service linking experienced amputees with newly disabled people, a panel of specialist legal firms and also a sports development service for disabled children and young people. The HelpBureau is available on 0845 230 0025.

LUPUS UK

St James House, Eastern Road, Romford RM1 3NH.
☎ 01708 731251.
@ headoffice@lupusuk.org.uk
Ⓦ www.lupusuk.org.uk

LUPUS UK provides information and support for people with lupus, or SLE, and their families both directly and through their network of self-help groups around the country. Publications include an information pack, a magazine and a range of other publications for individuals and professionals.

Macmillan Cancer Support

89 Albert Embankment,
London SE1 7UQ.
☎ 020 7840 7840 or 0808 800 1234 (Helpline). Textphone: 18001 0808 800 1234.
Ⓦ www.macmillan.org.uk

Macmillan Cancer Support is a major provider of cancer information and support. Specialist cancer nurses give information on any type of cancer or treatment, practical advice and details of local support groups and services. It publishes over 70 booklets and factsheets, has walk-in centres and a comprehensive website.

ME Association

7 Apollo Office Court, Radclive Road, Gawcott, Bucks MK18 4DF.
☎ 01280 818968.
Ⓦ www.meassociation.org.uk

The MEA represents the interests of and provides support and services to people with ME (myalgic encephalopathy), chronic fatigue syndrome and post viral fatigue syndrome. Information and support is available on the ME Connect Helpline

☎ 0870 444 1836.

Mencap

123 Golden Lane, London EC1Y 0RT.
☎ 020 7454 0454
Ⓦ www.mencap.org.uk

Advice & Information Service,
4 Swan Courtyard, Coventry Road, Birmingham B26 1BU.
☎ 0808 808 1111.
Textphone: 18001 0808 808 1111.
@ help@mencap.org.uk

Mencap Northern Ireland

Segal House, 4 Annadale Avenue, Belfast BT7 3JH.
☎ 028 9069 1351.

Mencap Cymru
Unit 31, Lambourne Crescent, Cardiff Business Park, Cardiff CF14 5GF.
☎ 029 2074 7588.

Mencap is the leading charity working with children and adults with learning disabilities in England, Wales and Northern Ireland. Mencap campaigns to ensure that people with a learning disability have the best possible opportunities to live as full citizens. It aims to influence new legislation and raise the profile of learning disability issues. It undertakes research into issues affecting people with a learning disability. Through its national network of more than 500 affiliated local societies Mencap offers local services, support and advice to people with learning disability and their parents/carers particularly in the areas of benefits, independent living, housing, education, employment and leisure activities. A range of literature is published including the newspaper Viewpoint.

Migraine Action

4th Floor, 27 East Street, Leicester
LE1 6NB.
☎ 0116 275 8317.
ⓦ www.migraine.org.uk

Migraine Action is an organisation for
people of all ages affected by migraine,
providing a link between them and
the medical profession. It provides
information, support groups, works
for improved services and monitors
research.

Mind

15-19 Broadway, London E15 4BQ.
☎ 0845 766 0163 (MindInfoLine) or
020 8519 2122.
@ contact@mind.org.uk
ⓦ www.mind.org.uk

Mind Cymru

3rd Floor, Quebec House, Castlebridge,
5-19 Cowbridge Road East, Cardiff
CF11 9AB.
☎ 029 2039 5123.

Mind is the leading mental health
charity in England and Wales. It offers a
telephone information line, publications
and support networks for users of
mental health services. Local Mind
associations (LMAs) provide a range of
services.
In Scotland, a similar organisation is:
Scottish Association for Mental Health,
Cumbrae House, 15 Carlton Court,
Glasgow G5 9JP.
☎ 0141 568 7000.
@ enquire@samh.org.uk
ⓦ www.samh.org.uk

Motor Neurone Disease Association

PO Box 246, Northampton NN1 2PR.
☎ 01604 250505.
@ enquiries@mndassociation.org
ⓦ www.mndassociation.org

The MNDA provides advice, support
and services for people with motor
neurone disease in England, Wales and
Northern Ireland and their families. It
issues a range of publications, employs
Regional Care Development Advisers,
has a network of local support groups
and offers help on specialist equipment.
Information is available on a Helpline
☎ 08457 62 62 62.

In Scotland contact:

Scottish Motor Neurone Disease Association

76 Firhill Road, Glasgow G20 7BA.
☎ 0141 945 1077.
@ info@mndscotland.org.uk
ⓦ www.scotmnd.org.uk

Multiple Sclerosis Society

MS National Centre, 372 Edgware Road,
London NW2 6ND.
☎ 020 8438 0700.
@ info@mssociety.org.uk
ⓦ www.mssociety.org.uk

Multiple Sclerosis Society Northern Ireland

The Resource Centre, 34 Annadale
Avenue, Belfast BT7 3JJ.
☎ 028 9080 2802.

Multiple Sclerosis Society Scotland
Ratho Park, 88 Glasgow Road, Ratho
Station, Newbridge EH28 8PP.
☎ 0131 335 4050.

Multiple Sclerosis Society Wales/ Cymru

Temple Court, Cathedral Road, Cardiff
CF11 9HA.
☎ 029 2078 6676

The MS Society provides information
and training centrally and also runs
several respite care centres. A range
of information and support services for
people with MS and those connected
with them are run through a network
of over 350 branches. The MS Helpline
offers advice and support Monday to
Friday, 9am-9pm on
☎ 0808 800 8000.

Muscular Dystrophy Campaign

61 Southwark Street, London SE1 0HL.
☎ 020 7803 4800.
@ info@muscular-dystrophy.org
ⓦ www.muscular-dystrophy.org

The Muscular Dystrophy Campaign focuses on neuromuscular conditions involving the weakening and/or wasting of muscles. Information and support on all aspects of life for children, adults and families living with any of these conditions can be provided in print, on the telephone or the information pages of its website. Regionally based staff provide practical advice and emotional support. A freephone Helpline is available on ☎ 0800 652 6352.

Myasthenia Gravis Association

1st Floor, Southgate Business Centre, Derby DE23 6UQ.
☎ 01332 290219.
@ mg@mga-charity.org
ⓦ www.mgauk.org

The Association has a network of local branches and Regional Organisers offering support to people with myasthenia gravis, which causes fluctuating muscle weakness, and information to those involved with them. Research is financed. A helpline is available on
☎ 0800 919922.

National Association for Colitis & Crohn's Disease

4 Beaumont House, Sutton Road, St Albans AL1 5HH.
☎ 0845 130 2233 (Information Line) or 01727 844 296. @ nacc@nacc.org.uk
ⓦ www.nacc.org.uk

NACC offers educational meetings, information and support to people living with Inflammatory Bowel Disease (IBD) both nationally and through 70 local groups.

National Association of Laryngectomee Clubs

Lower Ground Floor, 152 Buckingham Palace Road, London SW1W 9TR.
☎ 020 7730 8585.
ⓦ www.laryngectomy.org.uk

NALC has around 100 clubs throughout Britain and Ireland for people who have had their voice box removed. It also provides information in printed and other forms on living with a laryngectomy for patients, their families and carers.

National Autistic Society

393 City Road, London EC1V 1NG.
☎ 020 7833 2299.
@ nas@nas.org.uk
ⓦ www.autism.org.uk

NAS Northern Ireland

57A Botanic Avenue, Belfast BT7 1JL.
☎ 028 9023 6235.

NAS Scotland

Central Chambers
109 Hope Street, Glasgow G2 6LL.
☎ 0141 221 8090.

NAS Cymru

6-7 Village Way, Greenmeadow Springs Business Park, Tongwynlais,
Cardiff CF15 7NE.
☎ 029 2062 9312.

The National Autistic Society campaigns for rights and services for people with autism. It provides information to those affected by autism, support through a branch network, a parent-to-parent contact line, befriending schemes and also an education advocacy service. The NAS has developed the "EarlyBird" programme for newly diagnosed children and their parents. It has an extensive publications list and an Autism Helpline on 0845 070 4004.

National Blind Children's Society

Bradbury House, Market Street, Highbridge, Somerset TA9 3BW.
☎ 01278 764764.
@ enquiries@nbcs.org.uk
Ⓦ www.nbcs.org.uk

Family and Advice Support

2nd Floor Shawton House, 792 Hagley Road, Quinton, Birmingham B68 0PJ.
☎ 01278 764770.

NBCS provides information and a range of services for children with a visual impairment from birth to the end of formal education and their families including Family Support, Educational Advocacy, CustomEyes large print books, recreational activities and grants for home computers and specialist equipment.

National Deaf Children's Society

15 Dufferin Street, London EC1Y 8UR.
☎ /Textphone: 020 7490 8656.
@ ndcs@ndcs.org.uk
Ⓦ www.ndcs.org.uk

NDCS Northern Ireland

Wilton House, 5 College Square North, Belfast BT1 6AR.
☎ 028 9031 3170.
Textphone: 028 9027 8177.
@ nioffice@ndcsni.co.uk

NDCS Scotland

187-189 Central Chambers, 93 Hope Street, Glasgow G2 6LD.
☎ 0141 248 4457.
Textphone: 0141 222 4476.
@ ndcs.scotland@ndcs.org.uk

NDCS Wales Cymru

4 Cathedral Road, Cardiff CF11 9LJ.
☎ 029 2037 3474.
Textphone: 029 2023 2739.
@ ndcswales@ndcs.org.uk

NDCS campaigns for improved services for families with deaf children and provides impartial advice and support on all aspects of childhood deafness. A freephone Helpline is available on ☎/Textphone: 0808 800 8880 or @ helpline@ndcs.org.uk

National Eczema Society

Hill House, Highgate Hill, London N19 5NA.
☎ 020 7281 3553.
@ info@eczema.org Ⓦ www.eczema.org

The National Eczema Society provides a comprehensive information and advice service, an expanding network of local support groups, funds for research and a campaigning voice on behalf of people with eczema. Advice is available on a Helpline
☎ 0800 089 1122 (Monday-Friday 8am-8pm) or E helpline@eczema.org.

National Kidney Federation

The Point, Coach Road, Shireoaks, Worksop S81 8BW.
☎ 01909 544 999.
@ nkf@kidney.org.uk
Ⓦ www.kidney.org.uk

The NKF is run by and for kidney patients, working with associations of patients at individual renal units. It campaigns for improved treatment and support services and provides a wide range of information in print, through its website and by a telephone Helpline on ☎ 0845 601 0209.

National Society for Epilepsy

Chesham Lane, Chalfont St Peter, Bucks SL9 0RJ.
☎ 01494 601300.
Ⓦ www.epilepsynse.org.uk

NSE provides residential and medical services for adults with epilepsy in the UK. Residential care includes long and short term care, a high dependency unit, supported housing, and domiciliary care in community settings. NSE also provides specialist epilepsy training and information services, including websites, information resources and a Helpline on ☎ 01494 601400.

Parkinson's Disease Society

215 Vauxhall Bridge Road, London SW1V 1EJ.
☎ 020 7931 8080.
@ enquiries@parkinsons.org.uk
Ⓦ www.parkinsons.org.uk

The PDS provides support, advice and information to people with Parkinson's, their relatives and carers and campaigns to improve their quality of life. There are over 330 local branches and support groups around the UK.

A confidential helpline is available Monday-Friday 9.30am-9.00pm and Saturday 9.30am-5.30pm on
☎ 0808 800 0303.

Partially Sighted Society

7/9 Bennetthorpe, Doncaster DN2 6AA.
☎ 0844 477 4966.
@ info@partsight.org.uk

The Partially Sighted Society can provide information on all aspects of living with low vision, runs centres offering assessment for low vision aids in Exeter and Salisbury and has a number of local branches.

PINNT

PO Box 3126, Christchurch BH23 2XS.
Ⓦ www.pinnt.com

PINNT is a self-help organisation for people requiring intravenous, naso-gastric and other artificial nutrition therapy. It provides advice and mutual support through local groups. Half PINNT has been established for younger members and their parents and has its own section of the website.

The Prostate Cancer Charity

1st Floor, Cambridge House, 100 Cambridge Grove, London W6 OLE.
☎ 020 8222 7622.
@ info@prostate-cancer.org.uk
Ⓦ www.prostate-cancer.org.uk

In addition to raising awareness and supporting research, The Prostate Cancer Charity provides information and support to men with prostate cancer and their families. Information is available in print, on its website and in a DVD or video with sign language. A Helpline is available on weekdays and Wednesday evenings on
☎ 0800 074 8383.

Pulmonary Hypertension Association UK

Unit 3A, Enterprise Court, Farfield Park, Manvers, Rotherham S63 5DB.
☎ 01709 761450
@ office@phassociation.uk.com
Ⓦ www.phassociation.uk.com

PHA-UK aims to raise awareness of pulmonary hypertension and support those affected by the condition. They have regional support groups, a national conference, an internet chat room and a quarterly newsletter. Information can be provided on a Helpline
☎ 0800 389 8156.

REACH – The Association for Children with Hand or Arm Deficiency

PO Box 54, Helston, Cornwall TR13 8WD.
☎ 0845 130 6225.
@ reach@reach.org.uk
Ⓦ www.reach.org.uk

Reach aims to bring parents into contact with each other, giving them the opportunity to compare experiences and a means of understanding how others have coped or overcome problems. It can also provide information on what to do and where to go for advice regarding treatment for all types of deficiency, be it artificial limbs, appliances or surgery. It has branches in various parts of the country and offers a wide range of publications.

Restricted Growth Association
PO Box 1024, Peterborough PE1 9GX.
☎ 01733 759458 (Office and Helpline).
@ office@restrictedgrowth.co.uk
Ⓦ www.restrictedgrowth.co.uk

The RGA is a self-help organisation providing information and support to improve the quality of life for persons of restricted growth while encouraging and supporting their integration within the wider community. Communications are maintained through a quarterly magazine, a convention and regular social events. The Association has a network of Regional Co-ordinators with both a Full Adult Member of restricted growth and a Parent Member for each region.

Rethink
89 Albert Embankment, London SE1 7TP.
☎ 0845 456 0455.
@ info@rethink.org
Ⓦ www.rethink.org

Rethink works to help everyone affected by severe mental illness recover a better quality of life. It provides support with information, advice, services, groups, campaigns and research. Expert advice on issues affecting the lives of people living with mental illness is available from its National Advisory Service on 020 7840 3188 or advice@rethink.org

Royal National Institute of the Blind (RNIB)
105 Judd Street, London WC1H 9NE.
☎ 020 7388 1266.
@ helpline@rnib.org.uk
Ⓦ www.rnib.org.uk

RNIB Northern Ireland
40 Linenhall Street, Belfast BT2 8BA.
☎ 028 9032 9373.

RNIB Scotland
Dunedin House, 25 Ravelston Terrace, Edinburgh EH4 3TP.
☎ 0131 311 8500.

RNIB Cymru
Trident Court, East Moors Road, Cardiff CF24 5TD.
☎ 029 2045 0440.

RNIB is the country's largest charity promoting the rights and interests of, and providing services for, anyone with a sight problem. The range of services offered includes information, equipment, education, employment, leisure, talking books and advocacy. Information, support and advice is available from the RNIB Helpline
☎ 0845 766 9999 or @ helpline@rnib.org.uk

Royal National Institute for Deaf People (RNID)
19-23 Featherstone Street, London EC1Y 8SL.
☎ 020 7296 8000.
Textphone: 020 7296 8001.
@ informationline@rnid.org.uk
Ⓦ www.rnid.org.uk

RNID Northern Ireland
Wilton House, 5 College Square North, Belfast BT1 6AR.
☎/Textphone: 028 9023 9619.

RNID Scotland
Empire House, 131 West Nile Street, G1 2RX.
☎ 0141 341 5330.
Textphone: 0141 341 5347.

RNID Cymru

16 Cathedral Road, Cardiff CF11 9LJ.
☎ 029 2033 3034.
Textphone: 029 2033 3036.

The RNID aims for a better quality of life for the 9 million deaf and hard of hearing people through a combination of campaigning, raising awareness and providing information and services. Its interests include communications, education, employment, care services and equipment. It runs the Typetalk telephone relay service and carries out research and training. An information Helpline is available on ☎ 0808 808 0123. Textphone 0808 808 9000.

SANE

1st Floor, Cityside House, 40 Adler Street, London E1 1EE.
☎ 020 7375 1002.
@ info@sane.org.uk
Ⓦ www.sane.org.uk

SANE aims to raise awareness of mental illness, campaigns to improve services and initiates and funds research into the causes of serious mental illness. It also provides information and support to those experiencing mental health problems through its SANEline helpline, available 6pm-11pm every day on 0845 767 8000 or its SANEmail at sanemail@sane.org.uk

Scoliosis Association (UK)

4 Ivebury Court, 323-327 Latimer Road, London W10 6RA.
☎ 020 8964 5343.
@ sauk@sauk.org.uk
Ⓦ www.sauk.org.uk

SAUK is the national self-help support organisation for people with scoliosis (twisting or curving of the spine). It campaigns to raise awareness of scoliosis, provides opportunities for contact between families and teenagers who have had experience of scoliosis and

runs an information helpline on
☎ 020 8964 1166.

Scope

6 Market Road, London N7 9PW.
☎ 020 7619 7100
@ response@scope.org.uk
Ⓦ www.scope.org.uk

Scope is the disability organisation in England and Wales with a focus on people with cerebral palsy. It provides leaflets for parents, factsheets on therapies and aspects of living, carries out research and campaigns to achieve equality. For more information contact the Scope response Helpline, 9am-5pm weekdays on
☎ 0808 800 3333.

Sense – National Deaf-Blind and Rubella Association

101 Pentonville Road, London N1 9LG.
☎ 0845 127 0060.
Textphone: 0845 127 0062.
@ info@sense.org.uk
Ⓦ www.sense.org.uk

Sense Northern Ireland

The Manor House, 51 Mallusk Road, Mallusk, Co. Antrim BT36 4RU.
☎/Textphone: 028 9083 3430.

Sense Scotland

43 Middlesex Street, Kinning Park, Glasgow G41 1EE.
☎ 0141 429 0294.
Textphone: 0141 418 7170.

Sense Cymru

5 Raleigh Walk, Brigantine Place, Atlantic Wharf, Cardiff CF10 4LN.
☎ 0845 127 0090.
Textphone: 0845 127 0092.

Sense is a national charity that works with and campaigns for the needs of people who are deafblind. It provides information, advice and services for them, their families, carers and the professionals who work with them and also supports people who have sensory impairments with additional disabilities. Services include individual assessments, family support, a range of living options, day services and a holiday programme.

Sickle Cell Society
54 Station Road, London NW10 4UA.
☎ 020 8961 7795.
@ info@sicklecellsociety.org
Ⓦ www.sicklecellsociety.org

The Sickle Cell Society was formed in 1979 and works for improved services for people with sickle cell disorders and for a wider understanding of the condition. The Society, directly or through local support groups, provides a wide range of services from information, advice and counselling, to financial help, and an annual children's holiday.

Signature
Mersey House, Mandale Business Park, Belmont, Durham DH1 1TH.
☎ 0191 383 1155.
Textphone: 0191 383 7915.
@ durham@signature.org.uk
Ⓦ www.signature.org.uk

Signature Northern Ireland
Wilton House, 5 College Square North, Belfast BT1 6AR.
☎/Textphone 028 9043 8161

Signature Scotland
TouchBase Community Suite, 43 Middlesex Street, Glasgow G41 1EE.
☎ 0141 418 7191.
Textphone 0141 418 7193.

For information on services in Wales contact the Durham office above. Signature, the former Council for the Advancement of Communication with Deaf People (CACDP), undertakes the training, assessment and accreditation of interpreters using

British Sign Language and other forms of communication used by deaf people. It publishes an on-line directory of accredited Communication Professionals.

Speakability
1 Royal Street, London SE1 7LL.
☎ 020 7261 9572.
@ speakability@speakability.org.uk
Ⓦ www.speakability.org.uk

Speakability, registered as Action for Dysphasic Adults, supports people with aphasia and their carers as a result of stroke, head injury or other conditions resulting in a loss of communication skills without affecting intelligence. It also seeks to influence Government and other organisations to improve the level of services for people with aphasia and their carers. It provides a national network of support groups run by people with aphasia and an information service on Helpline ☎ 0808 808 9572.

Spinal Injuries Association
SIA House, 2 Trueman Place, Oldbrook, Milton Keynes MK6 2HH.
☎ 0800 980 0501 (Helpline) or 0845 678 6633.
@ sia@spinal.co.uk
Ⓦ www.spinal.co.uk

SIA supports spinal cord injured people and their families in England, Wales and Northern Ireland. It provides face-to-face support in Spinal Cord Injury Centres and through its Peer Support teams and gives information and advice through a telephone helpline, a website and a range of publications.

For Scotland contact:

Spinal Injuries Scotland
Festival Business Centre, 150 Brand Street, Govan, Glasgow G51 1DH.
☎ 0141 427 7686 or 0800 0132 305.
Ⓦ www.sisonline.org

Steps Charity Worldwide

Warrington Lane, Lymm, Cheshire
WA13 0SA.
☎ 0871 717 0044 (Helpline).
@ info@steps-charity.org.uk
Ⓦ www.steps-charity.org.uk

Steps supports those with a lower limb condition such as clubfoot or limb deficiency or a hip condition. It can provide publications, family contacts, a database of specialist doctors, an expanding website and a telephone helpline and information service.

Stroke Association

Stroke House, 240 City Road,
London EC1V 2PR.
☎ 020 7566 0300 or
0845 303 3100 (Helpline).
@ info@stroke.org.uk
Ⓦ www.stroke.org.uk

The Stroke Association provides UK-wide support for people who have had strokes, their families and carers while promoting research and campaigning to increase knowledge of stroke and improve stroke services. Community Services are available in many parts of the country including Communications Support, using volunteers with speech therapy support to improve the communication skills of people who have lost the ability to speak, read or write, and Family & Carer Support, providing skilled help to enable individuals and carers make the most of life after stroke. Over 500 Stroke Clubs are affiliated to the Stroke Association around England and Wales.

For local services in Northern Ireland and Scotland contact:

Northern Ireland Chest Heart & Stroke

21 Dublin Road, Belfast BT2 7HB.
☎ 028 9032 0184.
Ⓦ www.nichsa.com

Stroke Association Northern Ireland

Graham House, Knockbracken Healthcare Park, Saintfield Road, Belfast BT8 8BH.
☎ 028 9050 8020 (Helpline).
Ⓦ www.strokeni.org.uk

Chest, Heart & Stroke Scotland

65 North Castle Street, Edinburgh
EH2 3LT.
☎ 0845 077 6000 (Advice Line)
Ⓦ www.chss.org.uk

Terrence Higgins Trust

314-320 Gray's Inn Road, London
WC1X 8DP.
☎ 020 7812 1600.
@ info@tht.org.uk
Ⓦ www.tht.org.uk

THT campaigns to raise the public's awareness of HIV and improve the provision of services for people affected by HIV and those at risk from infection. Services are organised through regional centres in England, Scotland and Wales. It produces a range of publications and other material and provides information, advice and support on HIV-related topics such as treatment, support, welfare rights advice and counselling through its helpline THT Direct ☎ 0845 1221 200.

INDEX TO ADVERTISERS